THE RELAXED BODY BOOK
A High-Energy Anti-Tension Program

The Editors of
***American Health* Magazine**

**With
Daniel Goleman, Ph.D.,
and Tara Bennett-Goleman, M.A.**

Editor, Judith Groch
Photographs by Bill Hayward

Doubleday & Company, Inc.
Garden City, New York
1986

Editor Judith Groch
Design Will Hopkins, Ira Friedlander
Photography Bill Hayward
Managing Editor Kate Stuart
Copy Editor Fred Wiemer
Research Cathy Sears
Computer Services Gilbert Ferrer, Beth Schwaner
Editorial Assistant Kelly Vencill
Illustration Kimberly Belger-Suchocki
Art Staff Sandra McKee (administrator), Tim Boyse,
　　Robert Graf, Trish Marroquin
Consulting Editors Joel Gurin, T George Harris

EDITOR'S NOTE

BODYWATCH on PBS-TV. In the two years of work on this book with psychologist Daniel Goleman, Tara Bennett-Goleman, and others (see Acknowledgments), the editors of *American Health* magazine have at the same time been working on the new PBS-TV series, BODY-WATCH. The two projects have so enriched each other that video and print have, in this case, become sister media. Each speaks with unique force, but in harmony with the other.

That's because of a remarkable group of television people at WGBH-TV in Boston under David Ives. They're responsible for about one-third of all national prime-time PBS shows, including NOVA. For BODYWATCH, executive producer Christopher Gilbert and senior producer Laurie Donnelly brought together a brilliant research and production team. They showed such a grasp of physiological and medical research that the *American Health* editors and medical advisors sensed the chance for a first-rate series. The two groups worked together on the nine-part series, on the concurrent issues of the magazine, and on the book material as if they had been teamed up for 10 years. WGBH has even produced a special tape of relaxed body exercises for home video.

Because of BODYWATCH, millions of men and women are suddenly aware of the practical techniques described in this book, and know their value. More than 54% of all Americans now take exercise each week, and most learn that the body functions at its best when relaxed. Here's hoping the book helps you get into that high-energy state with ease and pleasure.
—T George Harris, Editor-in-Chief, *American Health Magazine*

ACKNOWLEDGMENTS

Our thanks go to the following experts and writers for material adapted for use in this book: Mark Bloom, Dianne Hales, Robert Hales, M.D., Hans Kraus, M.D., Lynne Lamberg, Perry London, Ph.D., James J. Lynch, Ph.D., Alexander Melleby, M.S., Mike Oppenheim, M.D., Paul Perry, Joann Ellison Rodgers, Carl Sherman, Richard D. Smith, Charles Spielberger, Ph.D., Carole Wade, Ph.D., and Kristin White.

We are also grateful to the body-work experts who have graciously supplied information and practical advice: Soleil Benmore, M.S., Andre Bernard, Roy Bonny, M.A., Judith Goleman Brod, M.A., Gail Fries, Kathy Harris, and Pat Ogden, M.A.

Finally, our special gratitude goes to Doubleday editor Loretta Barrett for her wise guidance—always relaxed, always on the mark.

Library of Congress Cataloging-in-Publication Data

The Editors of *American Health* Magazine;
Goleman, Daniel; Bennett-Goleman, Tara
The Relaxed body book.

Includes index.
1. Stress (Psychology)　2. Stress (Physiology)
3. Therapeutics, Physiological.　4. Relaxation
I. Goleman, Daniel.　II. Bennett-Coleman, Tara.
III. Groch, Judith.　IVB. American health (New York, N.Y.
BF575.S75R38 1986　613.7'9　85-20609
ISBN 0-385-19983-X
ISBN 0-385-19984-8 (pbk)

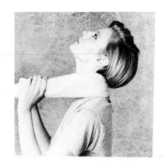

Contents

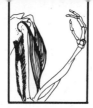

Part I: Relaxation: Mind and Body

Chapter 1

The Stress Spiral

Come, get, go, do;
hurry, hurry, hurry.

MIND-BODY CONNECTIONS

Remember these old-fashioned terms: frustration, hostility, worry, conflict, pressure, emotional trauma, alienation? Today this quaint collection has been superseded by that single portentous term with the hissing *s*'s—*stress*. In the media, in the research lab, on the job, and in the home, stress is everywhere, and everybody has it.

But what does it mean? In modern life, stress is often inevitable, even stimulating. Properly harnessed, it can fuel creativity and inspire accomplishment and success. But permitted to run amok, it also causes a variety of ills from headache and backache to emotional problems and serious biochemical disturbances.

This is a book about tense bodies. Its goal is practical and direct: to help you drain the tension from your body, to soothe and relax the physical ravages of both mental and physical stress. It is also, therefore, a book that deals with the mental and physical triggers that tie your body in knots. However, *The Relaxed Body Book*'s primary focus is physical (somatic) repair and prevention. It is not a book about coping with mental (cognitive) stress—dealing with the boss, your job, your family.

Each chapter of the book sets its tension problem within a broader context—physiological, psychological, or social—to give you the rationale behind its practical prescriptions. And unlike books devoted to a particular technique—yoga, stretches, massage, shiatsu, Alexander, Feldenkrais—*The Relaxed Body Book* explores the various disciplines to retrieve the best soothers for specific tension hot spots. Once you've brought calm and comfort to your body, we'll show you how to protect it from the return of tension.

The chapters in this book are divided into three sections. Part I, "Relaxation," deals with the nature of stress and the mind-body connections that participate in stress reactions.

In Part II you'll hit the "Tension Trail" and learn how to relax your head, face, jaw, neck, back, and feet. You'll also stop off at your digestive system where stress can create some very unpleasant gut reactions.

Part III, "Night and Day," visits the bedroom at day's end and then offers practical, everyday preventive measures to protect you from habits and situations that tie you in knots.

Within these divisions you'll find two types of chapters: There are straightforward ones that teach you how to relax your skeletal muscles—head, face, jaw, neck, back, feet. The source of stress in all of these cases may be either physical (working at a computer terminal) or mental (bracing your body as you deal with a difficult situation).

A second type of chapter focuses on internal systems that suffer physiologically when riven by mental or physical stress. These include a vulnerable cardiovascular system, an outraged gut, an ailing sex life, and sleep habits in shambles. Though these inner systems don't respond directly to stretches and massage, relaxation therapy and lifestyle changes are highly effective prescriptions.

Let's start by considering how these two types of stress gain a toehold in your body.

Psychological Stress

Mental stress is often associated with life's big-ticket disasters—major illness, divorce, job loss, or a death in the family. Yet it is also a product of the little insults of everyday life. As we move through the day juggling demands—Do it now; Fix it now; I forgot; Come, get, go; Hurry, hurry, hurry—tension ties both body and mind in knots. Studies show that these common hassles, rather than major crises, may eventually take a greater toll on health and well-being.

Consider life's small hassles: a misplaced key, a bounced check, a grumpy boss, a looming deadline. Any of these minor troubles is manageable when you're calm and relaxed—and a disaster when you're not. Often stress depends on how you see things. Is the overdrawn check a shameful embarrassment? Or will a simple phone call take care of it? How you construe the event makes all the difference. If you see it as a challenge, something you can handle, then it's not truly stressful. But if you let yourself feel overwhelmed, your body will be, too.

Once an event is seen as a threat, your body's stress reaction gets under way. First you become anxious and tense. After that each demanding moment in your day becomes that much more formidable. A person who's already anxious meets life's normal events as though they were crises. Pretty soon you find yourself stuck with the title role in the Book of Job.

As your stress level spirals upward, each minor mishap also adds to your physical level of tension. Your body stalls in a crisis mode, its tension levels escalating through the day. Stress may have its roots in mental reactions, but often its fruit is a tense body.

The body under threat harks back to those evolutionary fight-or-flight adaptations that have served it so well: The heart pumps faster and blood pressure rises to provide emergency blood supplies. The sweat glands increase secretion to toughen and coat the skin. Digestion slows so that blood can be diverted to the battlefront, and the liver manufactures more cholesterol, to provide additional energy resources. The muscles also do their part, tensing in readiness.

All this makes sense if there's a tiger lurking. Unfortunately, the emergency response is triggered by a primitive part of the brain that cannot distinguish between an advancing tiger and a meeting with saber-toothed accountants. What was once a life-saving mechanism now sets off that mark of modern life—garden-variety tension. Today's war zone is not the jungle, but your lower back and aching neck.

Physical Stress

Though psychological stress is the sophisticated angst of our times, let's not forget the simplest definition of stress is "pressure or strain." Stress—pure physical trauma—plays an important role in creating tense muscles. The body doesn't "care" whether muscle miseries derive from a job crisis or an uncomfortable chair. However, the physical trauma of modern automated life comes in subtle guise. A construction site looks dangerous; an office doesn't. Yet serious back injury may occur when a person, tethered all day to a work station, leans awkwardly from a chair to pick up a pencil. The intercom and computer terminal are as much a threat to soft, vulnerable bodies as the shovel and jackhammer are to the toughened hard hat.

BREAKING THE STRESS SPIRAL

Trying to understand and deactivate the mental and physical "stress spiral" before it sabotages your body brings us to the point of this book: You may not be able to stress-proof your life, but you can stress-guard your body.

The Relaxed Body Book will travel the head-to-toe tension trail undoing the physical imprints of mental and physical stress, soothing and relaxing your body's troubled spots. Individual chapters devoted to the body's prime stress targets offer therapeutic maneuvers you can do by yourself; no special equipment, such as biofeedback apparatus, is needed.

In the next chapter you'll find a self-test to help you rate and classify your reactions to stress. And you'll also learn to use the body scan to identify personal hot spots in which your body stores tension. With these diagnostic guides, you can work out a program of spot therapy—massage, stretches, and other muscle moves—plus overall relaxation techniques and work and lifestyle changes custom-designed for you.

And just as important, by enhancing your awareness of how you use your body, you'll develop an early-warning system to prevent tension—that chronically stiff neck or aching back—from returning regularly to blight your life.

The Anatomy of a Muscle Knot

The slow escalation of tension that can wind up in a knot of excruciating pain may begin innocently enough: A muscle tightens as it does in its usual activity. If you clench your fist, your forearm tenses; if you tighten your leg, your calf tightens. If you maintain the contraction, muscle tension will gradually build to the point where normally you have to relax.

A muscle is an incredible machine, its elastic fibers continually tensing and relaxing, shortening and lengthening as the muscle brings motion to your inert bones. But the contraction that ends in a knotted muscle is tensing gone beyond ordinary tightening into "bracing." The muscle contracts defensively, as though it were going to ward off an attack. Then the tension locks in, upsetting the usual delicate balance of tensing and relaxing that fine-tunes normal muscle moves.

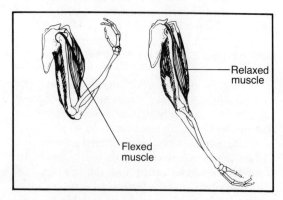

Relaxed muscle

Flexed muscle

Braced muscles are endlessly on battle alert. This sets off the process that may finally lock the muscle in a knot of pain, unable to relax. During contraction a healthy muscle produces metabolites, such as lactic acid, that must soon be flushed into the bloodstream. But if a contraction is held too long, the blood flow that nurtures the muscle is squeezed and waste by-products build up, causing pain. You can feel this process starting if you tense the muscle in your arm and hold the contraction. The dull throb that begins after a while signals the beginning of waste-product buildup. Keep it up, and the throb will become an outright ache.

The continued accumulation of waste products in a tense muscle sets up a vicious cycle: Pain triggers spasm, which further chokes off blood supply, causing a faster accumulation of irritating wastes. More pain.

This muscle-spasm cycle can be set off in many ways, but insults to your body are of two major types: The event may be physical (somatic) in origin or the stress trigger may be mental (cognitive).

Here's a *physical* example. If you change a light bulb in a ceiling fixture, you're likely to jam your head way back while you look up to see what you're doing. But your neck wasn't built for that extreme position.

The slight trauma to your neck muscles as you change the bulb may not seem like much, but it can produce mild discomfort in your neck. Without being consciously aware of it, you start hunching your shoulders slightly to avoid what seems a greater discomfort—straightening out your neck.

As the days pass, you may freeze in a hunch-shouldered stoop, your head still slightly tilted upward. That modest chin-up tilt makes you strain in another way: You now have to tense to see the world at eye level. This, in turn, puts more strain on the muscles at the back of your neck. These combined strains can slowly build into a neck ache so severe you can't move your head at all.

Now let's see how *mental* stress can tie you in knots. Watch someone who is late for an appointment driving a car in bad traffic. The shoulders hunch and the neck grows a bit shorter every time someone cuts in front or a light is missed. By the time the person finds a parking place, waits for an elevator stalled in the twilight zone, and rehearses excuses for being late, the victim's neck and shoulders may be a mass of knotted muscle.

Or suppose you are writing a difficult report that must be completed against a tight deadline. Your desk chair and typewriter are reasonably comfortable, so you can't blame them for what is about to happen.

As you sit there racing the clock, trying to concentrate and organize your material, you must still deal with the usual office obstacle course—phone calls, two-hour meetings, and assorted crises, including other deadlines "due yesterday."

Even though writing a report requires nothing but brainwork and a little finger action on the typewriter, your entire body—legs, arms, shoulders, neck, jaw, head—automatically braces for the mental challenge. As you write, your shoulders gradually rise toward your ears, freezing your neck at the same time. In fact, it's been said that most writers think with their shoulders. Your legs grow stiff as they wrap around the desk chair (after all, you might fall off the chair); your jaw clenches (must hang on to that last paragraph); and your forehead wrinkles (well, you're supposed to be thinking).

Now the telephone rings. You cradle the phone between your neck and an already tense shoulder and go on writing with your back pulled off center. Better tighten those legs, too. The clock ticks. You press on, leaning into your work. Now your back has no support and your jaw juts forward, yanking at your neck. Your stiff arms and hands are sending SOS signals, but your mind suppresses these and all other cries from an outraged body. Stand up and stretch for a while? Can't take the time!

You make the deadline. The report is a fine piece of work, but the tense, aching author is a pretzel. You may not feel it that night. But tomorrow there will be another report, and the painful collection of tense, abused muscles—you—that sits down to the next brilliant effort is already damaged goods. The eventual price may be chronic back trouble, tension headaches, jaw problems. And yet the origin of this muscular battering was mental, not physical.

By the time your ailing body rebels entirely, you may have forgotten about those reports—or the light bulb. You're frozen in pain and don't know how or why you got that way. All you want is relief—quickly.

Which brings us to how you can use this book to heal the incursions of stress and create a relaxed body.

HOT SPOTS

We each have a personal stress style. Two factors are involved: how we react to mental and physical triggers and where our bodies accumulate the ravages of stress. There's no universal pattern of mental and muscle tension, nor any standard package of antidotes that fits us all. Some people register mental stress in the gastrointestinal tract, while the rest of the body shows little sign of tumult; others get headaches when the pressure is on. And regardless of whether the stress trigger is mental or physical, those with a vulnerable back or neck will register the assault in those muscles. Often there are multiple triggers and varied trouble spots.

In the next chapter you will learn how to diagnose your primary stress style—mental, physical, or a bit of each. Once you have determined your "stress type," you should target your special stress repositories—neck, back, gut, feet—and then start with the body-soothing chapters that meet these urgent needs. After that, give the rest of your body a checkup. A relaxed body, after all, needs whole-body maintenance.

The first step is to know where your body needs immediate help. A nagging ache or pain may be obvious at this very moment. But consider, too, those trouble spots that may not be acting up just now. Where are they?

Your body has been telling you where it needs your attention for a long time: A simple inventory of the muscle aches that have plagued you over the last year or two will tell you where you need to concentrate. Have you had neck aches or backaches, foot cramps, repeated headaches? Is your stomach prone to butterflies? Do you get jaw aches? What spots have called out to you in their code of aches and pains? It may have happened once or twice a year—or just about every week. But the message is always the same: Pay attention to me.

RESOURCES—AND SOURCES

The stretches, massages, and soothers in this book have been drawn from a wide variety of techniques and then assembled in practical regimens for specific problems. Rather than adhering to a single school of body work, our guiding principle is to prescribe what's best for where you hurt. Listed below are some of the important techniques we especially wish to acknowledge and which you may wish to investigate further. If so, check the list of readings at the end of this book.

Swedish Massage
The most common system of massage in the United States today, Swedish massage was developed by Peter Henrik Ling early in the nineteenth century. Many of the basic muscle massages in the book are based on this approach.

Acupressure
This massage system, also known as "shiatsu," comes from the Orient. It uses acupuncture points throughout the body, but instead of needles, applies pressure to these points to produce many of the same effects. The advantages: No needles—and if you can reach these points, it's do-it-yourself therapy.

Yoga Exercises
Yoga exercises combine stretching, relaxation, deep breathing, and concentration. Each yoga position is designed to bring awareness to a specific area of the body as muscles are stretched and then relaxed.

Ideokinesis

Movement involves the mind as well as the body. Ideokinesis uses this intimate link to correct the way the body moves. Mabel Todd, a movement educator at Columbia University, developed this method, which uses guiding images to coax the body into movement that best fits its anatomy. For example, imagine your head is filled with helium, lifting and lengthening your spine.

The Alexander Technique

In the early 1900s Frederick M. Alexander, an actor, developed a method of postural reeducation to help people learn more efficient, stress-free ways of using the body. The key, said Alexander, is to lift the head and neck properly. This technique is popular with many dancers and actors.

The Feldenkrais Technique

Developed by the late Israeli physicist Moshe Feldenkrais, this method integrates movements in a natural flow that alleviates stress and leads to increased grace and energy. Feldenkrais workers tackle many stress ailments with a gentle system aimed at teaching people to reeducate their body's movement habits.

PREVENTION: STAYING PAIN-FREE

If you're prone to aches that keep coming back—a tension headache, say, or an aching neck or back—then preventive measures are in order.

Throughout this book you'll find a range of methods that will help you head off pain before it starts. These protective moves aim at changing the habits that reknit the knots.

Because a recurrent muscle ache may originate in a habitual way of holding or moving part of your body, some of the preventive techniques are designed to reprogram your movement patterns. You'll take a fresh look at how you move, and practice alternatives that won't cause tension.

Stretches can also avert muscle knots. For many areas of the body you'll find sets of stretches designed to lengthen muscle fibers— a direct antidote to the fiber-shortening that may eventually lead to spasm.

A final preventive measure is to enhance your awareness of trouble spots. The more sensitive you are to the state of your muscles, the more likely you are to notice early signs of tension. In each section you'll find techniques designed to sensitize you to those crucial muscles.

And so with this book in hand you are ready to go to work: to discover and befriend your body; to learn "muscle talk," a two-way language; and to short-circuit the stress spiral. Your goal—to enjoy the physical and emotional benefits of a Relaxed Body.

The Quick Fix

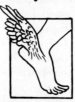

When a muscle is locked in spasm, you need quick relief. Throughout this book you will find suggestions marked by a quick-fix symbol. This feature lets you zero in on things you can do *right now* to ease pain.

Usually, these will be techniques that get blood flowing through knotted muscles: heat applications, massages, and simple movements that stimulate blood circulation so it carries off pain-causing toxins.

Heat is effective first aid because it tricks the body's thermostats into increasing blood flow to the heated area. This temperature adjustment is part of the natural mechanism that cools the body. But muscles benefit because increased blood flow clears out toxic buildup and breaks the pain-tension spiral.

Massage acts in a slightly different way. It, too, produces healing heat, but it also seems to work more directly, triggering nerves to send a message to the brain to relax the muscle.

Gentle movement, like heat and massage, can help untie a muscle knot by speeding blood flow, but it can also ease the strangled muscle into the relaxed state it assumes during normal movements.

Depending on the location and structure of the ailing muscle, these remedies—heat, massage, movement—will be recommended as quick fixes for pain.

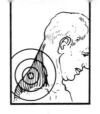

Chapter 2

Tension
Targets

To befriend your body,
learn "muscle talk"—
a two-way language.

You are now ready to learn to use certain basic tools that relax you even as they help you find your tension hot spots.

Because chronic tension becomes such a muscular habit, the feeling may eventually seem normal. One of the first steps in developing a relaxed body is to rediscover what it feels like to be relaxed all over, much like a soft, floppy baby. Several techniques presented here—progressive relaxation, the body scan, autogenic suggestion, meditation—are designed to induce this state of total flop.

But it's not enough to inspect your body. Since so often physical tension is mind-driven, it's important to determine your personal stress style—mental, physical, or both. Once you know that, you'll be ready to develop a daily routine tailored to the individual way your body reacts to stress.

Let's start with basic techniques.

PROGRESSIVE RELAXATION

One widely used method is "progressive relaxation," since it progresses through the body relaxing each major muscle area. The technique—or something very much like it—is also called "deep-muscle relaxation."

By any name, the strategy is the same: You methodically sweep through your body, learning what each muscle group feels like when it's tense, then when it's relaxed. Your aim is to leave those muscles in a deeply relaxed state. This technique was pioneered by a physician, Edmund Jacobson, who wrote a book in 1929 with the ironic title *You Must Relax*. Since then progressive relaxation has been used widely to help people fight stress.

A most important lesson to be learned from progressive relaxation is the fundamental difference between being relaxed and being tense. Once you can tune in to your muscles, you may choose to use the muscle scan (see p. 13), a quicker and less cumbersome relaxer. But the scan works best after you have mastered progressive relaxation.

The irony of Dr. Jacobson's title, of course, is that you can't make an effort to relax—you have to *let* it happen. At the muscular level that means you allow the fibers of the muscle to lengthen—relax. Progressive relaxation does just that.

But it has another benefit: As you sweep through your body, you have a chance to study the messages of muscle tension. You'll learn to sense the difference between relaxation and tension. Once you can tune in to these signals, you can use them to release tension whenever you sense a hot spot in the making.

It's best to practice progressive relaxation diligently, a session a day, until you've mastered it. Then return to it from time to time for a refresher. Once you've mastered progressive relaxation, it can be applied to the body-scan technique and will be useful in heading off tension no matter what you're doing.

How to Do Progressive Relaxation

The first few times you practice, read a section, do it, then read ahead. Pretty quickly, you'll be soloing. Or you may wish to listen to a tape (see Resources, p. 189).

Find a comfortable, firm surface—a plush rug or exercise mat. A bed is too soft. Lie on your back, your arms extended along your sides, your feet comfortably apart. Loosen any tight clothes, and take your shoes off.

Begin by tensing all the muscles in your body, from head to toe. Tense your hands and arms, clench your jaws, feel the tightness in your chest and stomach, your back, legs, and feet. Hold the tension while you sense the overall feeling of strain and tightness throughout your body. Now take a breath, hold it, and exhale as you relax and let go. Ahhhh. . . . Sense the relief as you relax, and note the calm in your body as you stop tensing.

From here on, concentrate on each tension spot individually. The basic principle is to tense one part of your body while keeping the rest relaxed. Hold the tension in each part for a few seconds, long enough to get a firm idea of what it feels like. Then breathe deeply, hold your breath for a moment, and let go of the tension as you breathe out.

Make your *hands* into fists. As you clench them, feel the tension in your hands and arms. Relax and let go. . . . Press your *arms* down on the surface below you and feel the tension running through them up into the shoulders—hold it—relax and let go. . . . Make a muscle in your arm, bending it up toward your shoulder—hold—release, let go, and relax. Let your arm drop back down, free of tension . . . relaxed and soft. Now the other arm.

Next, shrug your *shoulders* up toward your ears. Feel the tension in your neck and shoulders—hold—relax and let go. Feel your shoulders drop down to a relaxed position, free of tension. Now shrug your left shoulder up toward your ear—hold—relax and let go. Now your right—hold—and let go. Feel the relaxation spreading up through your arms and shoulders.

Wrinkle your *forehead*—feel the tension—relax and let go. Let your forehead be smooth and relaxed. Now scrunch your *eyes* tight shut—hold—and let go. Stretch your *mouth* open as wide as you can—hold it—and let your mouth close gently. Clench your *jaws*, gripping with your teeth—hold—and release. Your mouth will now be free of tension, your teeth apart, your lips closed gently, or open a bit—your whole face resting easy. Feel the tension dissolve from your face . . . your forehead relaxed, your eyes relaxed, your mouth and jaws relaxed, easy, soft. . . . Feel the softness spreading through your face, neck, shoulders, arms.

Fill your *lungs* with a big, deep breath, and hold it while you explore the tension in your chest. Now let go and let your breathing be free and natural, your chest relaxed. Next, suck in your *stomach* and hold it, feeling the tension. Let go; feel the tension ease up. Now arch your *back*, as though you had a pillow under it—hold—relax and ease back down . . . relax and let go. Feel the sense of ease spreading through your whole upper body . . . breath free and easy . . . your face at ease . . . neck free of tension . . . your shoulders and arms relaxed . . . chest and stomach soft and relaxed . . . back sinking into the surface beneath . . . your whole upper body soft and easy.

Now tighten your *buttocks and hips* and press your legs and heels against the surface beneath—hold—and let go . . . relax . . . . Feel your *legs* soften . . . now curl your *toes* down, pointing away from your knees—hold—release and let go. Bend your toes back up toward your knees—hold—relax and let go.

Let yourself become more and more relaxed each time you breathe out. Feel your whole body floating free . . . soft . . . relaxed . . . the tension slipping away . . . your face relaxed . . . neck relaxed . . . arms and shoulders soft . . . stomach, chest, back at ease. . . . Feel this lovely, relaxed state spread through your whole body, a wave of soft warmth. . . .

Spend several minutes feeling deeply peaceful and relaxed. When you're ready to get up, do it slowly, sitting up first, then standing. As you go about your day, remember this calm, peaceful state of relaxation.

THE WHOLE-BODY SCAN: TUNING IN TO TROUBLE SPOTS

Though it's useful to do this full-scale relaxation exercise, it's also important to give your body quicker, more frequent checkups aimed at detecting the start of tension buildup. Most people are unaware of tension creep. It goes on subtly and silently until you are suddenly jarred into noticing pain signals. The whole-body scan, below, will help increase your sensitivity to tension pockets, lower your overall stress level, and short-circuit trouble before it gets out of hand.

The body scan is a kinesthetic equivalent of checking out your appearance in a mirror. But instead of a visual survey, quiet awareness of internal sensations is used to monitor muscle-tension patterns in major areas of the body. Though slow at first, it will take but a few moments once you're familiar with the routine. The scan is related to the progressive-relaxation technique you've just learned, but instead of exploring the tensed-relaxed contrast, it teaches you to inspect your muscles and decode their messages.

Once you become adept at scanning, you can use the technique any time your body needs a quick tension review or you feel an overall need to calm down. And the more you practice the scan, the more surely you'll be able to zero in on your usual tension-storage zones. If you're a jaw clencher or a neck tensor, a scan can target those areas regularly and then go on to check other aches in the making.

13

After you've mastered the scan, particularly its fast or target versions, you should turn to it throughout the day as a quick "relaxercise."

You may wish to use reminders—events that come up repeatedly during the day—as your cue to scan your body. For example, you could do a quick scan every time you hang up the phone or whenever you wait for an elevator. If you're at school, the bells at the end of class are a natural reminder. Another cue can be sitting down for a meal (see "Mindful Eating," p.119). And, of course, there's always the peace and quiet of the bathroom.

Like the progressive-relaxation routine, while you're learning the scan, simply read over these instructions, go as far as you can from memory, then read the next section—and on through the whole scan. Or you may wish to use a tape (see Resources, p.189).

During practice sessions, protect yourself from distractions. Find a room with little or no background noise, where you can be alone. If possible, have someone else answer the phone or door, watch the kids, or deal with little problems. And don't practice when you're drowsy—say, right after a meal or before bedtime. The idea is to stay alert.

Most important: Give yourself plenty of time to do the scan slowly and carefully. Don't try it when you're rushed or just about to go off for an appointment. Try to find a break in your schedule when you have open time, so you can feel more relaxed.

How to Scan

Wear comfortable clothes and lie on your back on the floor, on a soft but firm surface—a thick rug, exercise pad, or blanket. (Once you have learned the technique, you can do it in any position.) Let your feet spread several inches apart and your arms fall to your sides. Find the most natural position for you. The scan uses the power of your attention to bring a soothing awareness to your body's tension spots. Now close your eyes and bring your attention to your breath. Notice very carefully how your breath *feels*. Don't try to control your breathing—just become keenly aware of the feeling.

You might notice how your stomach and chest rise and fall with each breath. Note the cool flow of air into your nose and the warm flow back out again. Or you may observe the sensation of air flowing into and filling your lungs as your chest expands, then its outward rush as you exhale and your chest falls. You may find your breath uneven on the in-breath and out-breath, or the rhythm may be smooth and regular. There may be a slight pause between inhaling and exhaling.

Whatever you find is fine. Just be aware of these sensations.

On each inhalation, scan a muscle area. On each exhalation, try to release any tension you feel. It's simple: As you become aware of tension in a muscle area, think about that tension slipping away as you exhale. Imagine each exhalation as emptying your body of tension. Stay with each muscle area for a long, still moment. Work on it through several in- and out-breaths. Don't hurry. If you have more tension in one area, linger as long as you wish.

It doesn't matter exactly what you feel in each area—warmth, tingling, pressure, stiffness, or nothing in particular. All that matters is that you focus awareness on each area, and keep it there while you scan for tension and mentally release whatever you find.

Don't worry if your mind wanders while you're scanning. Just bring your attention back to the last point in the scan and continue.

Now bring your awareness to your *head and face*. Tour your whole head with your mind's eye—your scalp, the back and sides of your head, your forehead and temples, eyes and nose, cheeks and mouth, jaw and chin. Take plenty of time.

Give each area a careful survey. Observe any sensations you find there as you breathe in, and imagine any tension there melting away as you breathe out. On every in-breath, scan; on every out-breath, release. Feel the tension slipping away as you exhale. . . .

Now focus on your *neck, shoulders, and arms*. Scan the front and back of your neck, move to your shoulders, then slowly down each arm to your hands. Take plenty of time, especially in your neck and shoulders. Wherever you feel tension, stay with it for a while, scanning on the in-breath, releasing on the out-breath. Feel a deepening relaxation as you move through your tension spots, relaxing the tightness, leaving the muscles soft, heavy, and warm. . . .

Move on to your *chest and stomach*. Notice how they rise and fall with each breath. Be sure to let your stomach rise and fall as you breathe, not just your chest. Feel the tension slip away with each breath, your chest getting more relaxed, your stomach softer and fuller. Breathe—in, out—more and more relaxed, deeper and deeper. . . .

Now scan your *back*, from shoulders to buttocks. Don't rush; there's a lot to notice here. Is your back stiffly arched or relaxed? With each in-breath, find a spot in this vast territory and concentrate on sensations. With each out-breath, imagine the tension draining away. Feel your back pressing down onto the surface beneath. As you release the tension, let your back sink down more deeply and fully. . . . Breathe, relax.

Next, your *legs and feet*. Scan each leg down through the foot—don't forget the sole. Feel whatever sensations you find there and relax away the tension. Scan and relax, scan and relax.

Now just let yourself lie limp while you scan up and down your whole body. Whenever you come to a spot of tension, spend some time there, breathing out the tension, relaxing it away. . . .

Without moving, just lie there and open your eyes. While your eyes stare off into space, notice what it's like to be completely relaxed, yet alert and aware.

When you're ready to get up, take a few deep breaths, and get up slowly, in stages. Keep this feeling of relaxation with you as you return to your daily activities. Remember, there's always another scan.

The Quick Scan

Once you've learned to do the whole-body scan, you can turn to it whenever you have a few free moments to drain the tension from your body or feel a need to relax—before a big interview or when you're nervous, angry, or frightened.

You can scan no matter what position your body is in—sitting, standing, lying down. But it's better if you are still and if you can withdraw your attention totally from everything else for a few moments.

In the quick form, spend just a few breaths on each major area:

- head and face
- neck and shoulders
- stomach and chest
- upper back, lower back, and buttocks
- legs and feet

Wherever you find tension building, spend more time. But be sure to complete the scan.

The Superquick Scan

You do this one in the time it takes for three deep breaths. On the first breath, scan your head and shoulders as you breathe in, and relax them as you breathe out. On the second breath, scan from your shoulders to the top of your legs on the in-breath, and release the tension there on the out-breath. And on the third, do the same for your legs and feet. You can do the whole thing while you're waiting for a red light to turn green.

The Target Scan

If you're prone to tension in a particular spot, zero in on that area. If it's your shoulders, for example, just take a breath or two to scan your shoulders, then spend as much time as you can scanning and relaxing, scanning and relaxing, as you breathe in and out.

Some Tips

- Eventually, you may develop your own menu of hot spots and your own favorite route through your body. Good. Some people can expand their awareness so they scan the whole body at once. That's fine, too, though not a necessary goal.

■ Don't let yourself take shortcuts that tune out certain areas of your body. Every few days or weeks, take the time for an extended, careful scanning session, just to be sure you're not missing something.

■ Enjoy the scan. Let your mind be absorbed in the full sensory exploration of your body. Don't worry about results. However you feel at the end of the scan is fine. The results will come gradually, but surely, if you keep at it.

AUTOGENIC SUGGESTION

Autogenic training—*self*-regulation—is a technique that uses the power of the mind to control those inner automatic body systems—heartbeat, breathing, blood pressure—that create the fight-or-flight stress response. Developed by two physicians, Johannes Schultz and Wolfgang Luthe, the technique uses verbal cues to condition your body to reduce stress reactions. The goal is rhythmic breathing, a calm heartbeat, and warmth and heaviness in the limbs, suggesting increased blood flow to those areas. Here's a brief version of how to go about it. (For a tape to guide you, see Resources, p.189.)

Make yourself comfortable in an armchair that supports your head and arms, or lie down but support your neck with pillows. Eventually, you'll be able to use this technique in odd moments of the day—lunch or coffee break—but in your early practice sessions it's best to allow sufficient time, perhaps at the end of the day. Loosen any tight clothing, close your eyes, and focus your attention on your breathing.

Imagine your breathing rolling in and out with the rhythm of ocean waves. Say to yourself, "My breathing is calm and effortless . . . calm and effortless. . . ."

As you breathe, imagine waves of relaxation flowing over your body . . . moving through your chest and shoulders, into your arms and back muscles . . . downward into your hips and legs. With each breath, try to feel waves of heaviness and warmth filtering into your arms and legs.

Feel a tranquil sense of relaxation moving through your body. Everything is heavy . . . peaceful.

Now focus on your *arms and hands* and say to yourself: "Warmth and heaviness are flowing into my arms and hands. My right arm is heavy and warm; my left arm is heavy and warm. Warmth is flowing into my arms and gently down into my wrists, hands, and fingers. It feels relaxed and pleased."

Feel your whole body relax as the warmth flows into your hands. All your worries are departing, all cares are forgotten . . . let go . . . let go. All thoughts are draining from your mind. Focus on the pleasant, relaxed feeling.

If thoughts intrude, don't worry. Just send them away gently and concentrate on: "My arms are getting heavy and warm. Warmth is flowing . . . flowing."

While your arms grow heavy and warm, check for tension elsewhere in your body. Is your jaw loose and are your eyelids gently closed? You're becoming very relaxed and limp.

Now focus on your *legs*. Touch them to make you aware of them. Heaviness and warmth are moving down from your arms to your legs. Focus on the feeling.

As the warmth spreads, silently say to yourself: "My legs are becoming heavy and warm. Warmth is flowing into my feet . . . into my toes. Everything is heavy and warm, pleasantly warm. . . ."

Now focus on all your limbs and be aware how heavy, warm, and limp they've become. Silently: "My arms and legs are so heavy and warm. . . . Muscles everywhere are letting go, letting go . . . I'm becoming more and more relaxed."

Take a deep breath and focus on the feeling of air filling your lungs. Breathe deeply down into your abdomen. Breathe out and say, "I am calm." Breathe deeply and again say, "I am calm . . . I am calm."

At first, say these words only when you are deeply relaxed, but with practice you will be able to relax yourself by simply thinking, "I am calm." If your day is a disaster—the computer is down or you're caught in traffic—this potent phrase will summon these deeply relaxed feelings. Practice until it's automatic.

When your practice session is over, lie there and realize that you can bring about this pleasant, safe sense every time you do these exercises. Now count to three and take a deep breath with each number. Open your eyes (unless you are trying to fall asleep). Notice that you are peaceful, relaxed, yet alert.

Before returning to everyday activities, yawn and stretch; shake your hands briskly.

THE RELAXATION RESPONSE

Meditation is an all-round relaxer that soothes both mental worries and physical tension. It's so effective that physicians and psychologists prescribe it regularly for people with stress-related problems, such as high blood pressure, chronic pain, and certain digestive disorders. Though it's not a cure-all, it's a good supplement to other treatments.

At first, researchers attributed meditation's benefits to the "relaxation response," a state of especially deep relaxation that may occur during meditation. In this state muscles relax, breathing slows, and blood pressure drops. But subsequent research has found the relaxation it induces is no different from that of other techniques, such as progressive relaxation. Dr. Herbert Benson, associate professor of medicine at Harvard, explains that most scanning and visualizing techniques provide different routes to the same experience—the relaxation response. Many people, however, prefer meditation to other forms of relaxation, perhaps because it takes your mind off your worries at the same time it relaxes your body.

To see whether meditation is your cup of tea, try it for about ten days. Work it into your daily routine for fifteen to twenty minutes each day, at any convenient time. Just try to be regular. (If you would like tape instruction, see Resources, p.189.) Here are some tips before you start:

■ Don't meditate after eating a heavy meal or at other times when you're drowsy, such as right before bed.

■ Sit upright in a comfortable, straight-backed chair. There's no need to torture your knees in a yogic pretzel—but don't sit in a plush easy chair either. The idea is to stay alert, not doze off.

■ No disturbances. Try to arrange things so you won't have to answer the phone, mind the kids, or otherwise stop in the middle.

■ Loosen any tight clothing, such as belts; take your shoes off.

■ Stay with it. Commit yourself to a specific length of time, preferably fifteen to twenty minutes, and don't let a sudden distraction ruin your session. Set a timer (nothing too loud or jarring) or glance at a clock to check the time. But don't stop till your time is up.

How to Meditate

Sit comfortably in your chair and focus on your breath as it comes and goes through your nostrils. Pay attention to each breath—the full inhalation, the full exhalation. Whenever your mind wanders, just bring it back to your breath.

Don't try to control your breathing. If it gets faster, let it; if it slows, fine. Just continue to be *aware* of it.

If you hear distracting sounds, notice some sensation in your body, or if your mind wanders, bring it back to your breath.

Try to be aware of the feeling of breathing: the subtle play of air moving through your nose or on your upper lip, or anything that strikes you. But stay completely focused on your breath.

If your mind wanders, try counting your breaths. On the in-breath, count "one," on the out-breath, count "two," and so on, up to ten. Then start over again.

WHAT'S YOUR STRESS STYLE?

Once you've mastered these basic relaxation techniques and highlighted your body's specific hot spots, it's time to match your unique stress style to overall antidotes designed to relax both body and mind. Remember, the source of muscle tension may be awkward muscle moves and unfriendly furniture, but it's just as likely to be mentally fueled. Your daily routine should therefore include a stress defuser that will serve as an overriding inoculation against life's hassles.

But people differ not only in how they experience stress but in the kind of therapy they feel comfortable with. Before choosing your all-purpose stress antidote, it's useful to determine your personal stress type. The simple test below will help you establish this profile so you can then choose your relaxation therapy accordingly. Remember, there's a distinction between stress targets in your body and your principal way of *reacting* to stress. The target of stress can be a bodily or somatic change—tense muscles, constricted arteries, digestive uproar, even trouble in the brain's sleep center. However, your personal stress style is the overall all-too-familiar way you react.

There are three basic stress types—primarily physical, mainly mental, or a mixture.

Physical stress types feel tension in the body—jitters, butterflies, the sweats. Mental types experience stress mainly in the mind—worries and preoccupying thoughts. Mixed types react with both responses in about equal measure. Though your goal is to deal with the physical targets, you may wish to take your profile into account when choosing a relaxer.

Take the quick test below to help you find your type.

Stress Style: Body, Mind, Mixed?

When you're feeling anxious, what do you typically experience? Check all that apply:
- ☐ 1. My heart beats faster.
- ☐ 2. I find it difficult to concentrate because of distracting thoughts.
- ☐ 3. I worry too much about things that don't really matter.
- ☐ 4. I feel jittery.
- ☐ 5. I get diarrhea.
- ☐ 6. I imagine terrifying scenes.
- ☐ 7. I can't keep anxiety-provoking pictures and images out of my mind.
- ☐ 8. My stomach gets tense.
- ☐ 9. I pace up and down nervously.
- ☐ 10. I'm bothered by unimportant thoughts running through my mind.
- ☐ 11. I become immobilized.
- ☐ 12. I feel I'm losing out on things because I can't make decisions fast enough.
- ☐ 13. I perspire.
- ☐ 14. I can't keep worrisome thoughts out of my mind.

Stress-Style Scoring

Give yourself a Body point for each of these: 1, 4, 5, 8, 9, 11, 13.

Give yourself a Mind point for each of the following: 2, 3, 6, 7, 10, 12, 14.

If you have more Mind than Body points, consider yourself a mental stress type. If you have more Body than Mind points, your stress style is physical. About the same number of each? You're a mixed reactor.

Caution: When Relaxing Is Unrelaxing

A handful of people get even more tense when they try to relax. The symptoms of relaxation-induced tension are various: restlessness, headache, feeling uptight or upset to the point of crying, rapid breathing, sweating, or tremors. These are also the standard symptoms of anxiety. In a study at the State University of New York at Albany, about half the people starting meditation and a third doing deep-muscle relaxation experienced mild forms of these symptoms. And a few people had more intense reactions.

One cause seems to be that people aren't used to the new sensations—floating, heaviness, tingling or numbness—that often accompany states of relaxation. Habitual levels of tension have become so familiar and comfortable that one feels strange when they start to go.

The anxiety, one theory holds, is a reaction to these unfamiliar sensations. Indeed, some people get a bit panicked at the sense of "losing control" associated with letting go of the tension that armors their body. And for some hard-driving types, the idea of taking time to "do nothing"—that is, relax—may be too threatening.

Whatever the cause, if a relaxation method makes you more tense, try some adjustments. One is to stop doing it for a while, then go back to it gradually. Another is to shift to a different technique. Someone who panics at muscle relaxation may love meditation, or vice versa.

CHOOSING A RELAXER

Knowing your stress type will guide you in selecting the kind of overall relaxer that should work best for you. The idea is to match your stress style to an activity that counters it directly. You may want to experiment with several possiblities. Be certain to pick something you really enjoy. The signs that you've hit upon the right relaxer are simple: You should look forward to the activity, enjoy it while you do it, and feel more relaxed afterward.

Body

If stress registers mainly in your body, you'll need a remedy that will break up the physical stress pattern. This may be a vigorous body workout, but a slow-paced, even lazy muscle relaxer may be equally effective. Here are some suggestions to get you started:
Aerobics
Calisthenics
Swimming
Biking
Rowing
Working out
Walking
Yoga
Massage
Soaking in a hot bath, sauna

Mind

If you experience stress as an invasion of worrisome thoughts, the most direct intervention is anything that will engage your mind completely and redirect it—meditation, for example. On the other hand, some people find the sheer exertion of heavy physical exercise unhooks the mind wonderfully and is fine therapy:
Meditation
Autogenic suggestion
Reading
Crossword puzzles
TV, movies
Games like chess or cards
Knitting, carpentry, and other handicrafts
Any absorbing hobby
Vigorous exercise

Body/Mind

If you're a mixed type, you may want to try a physical activity that also demands mental rigor:
Competitive sports (racquetball, tennis, squash, volleyball, etc.)
Meditation
Any combination from the Mind and Body lists

Remember, there are no hard and fast rules for choosing a relaxer. Mind and body are so tightly linked that some body reactors do better with a mental relaxer and some mind reactors say the same about body techniques.

The stress-style test is a guideline only, perhaps most helpful to people who have not yet built a relaxer into their daily routine. Being aware of your stress style may help you understand your preference for certain activities and encourage you to experiment with others perhaps better suited to your needs.

Now, equipped with some specific relaxation techniques and an awareness of your body's tension targets, it is time to hit the tension trail.

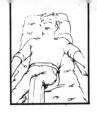

Chapter 3

The Heart of the Matter

Cultivate the lifesaving graces—slow down, relax, listen, and laugh.

This book is designed to travel the tension trail from head to toe, but before we set forth, it makes sense to pause at that great hardworking muscle—the heart. We've been talking about the physical toll of mental stress; clearly, the heart is the central target for a stress-driven, unrelaxed way of life. Your shoulders will survive the incursions of tension; your heart may not. And yet the heart itself is not meant to be relaxed; its job is to pump away efficiently all the days of your life. But the biochemical changes brought about by stress and tension can erode vital blood vessels—the lifelines to the heart itself and the body beyond.

So one obvious reason to pursue a relaxed body is to control the mind-driven physical reactions that etch themselves upon the cardiovascular system. An obvious place to start is with so-called Type A behavior. Even if you're not a true Type A, the paradigm is useful in gaining an understanding of how one important type of mental stress can devastate so sturdy an organ. From there we can move on to some techniques designed to defuse unrelaxed—and potentially dangerous—behavior.

TYPE A: HOSTILE, HARRIED, HARD-DRIVING

In 1959 San Francisco cardiologists Meyer Friedman and Ray Rosenman noted a characteristic type of behavior among heart-attack patients. They dubbed it "Type A," as opposed to "Type B" behavior. Type A's, they proposed, are deeply competitive, harried, hostile, and always racing the clock. They live in a dog-eat-dog world where mistrust makes it impossible to relax and lean on others. Type A's in their studies were twice as likely to have a heart attack as the more laid-back, trusting Type B's, even when factors such as cholesterol and smoking were discounted.

The Type A link to heart attacks has evolved as an ongoing medical debate, and 1985 studies have added fuel to the controversy. For example, a major multicenter study headed by Dr. Robert B. Case of New York's St. Luke's–Roosevelt Hospital Center has found that among people who've had a heart attack, Type A's are no more likely to have a second, fatal attack than Type B's. And at the University of Texas, researchers tracked 3,110 high-risk men and found that among those who eventually did have a heart attack, Type A or Type B behavior made no difference. On the other hand, at Mt. Zion Medical Center in San Francisco and Stanford University a new study of 1,013 heart-attack patients found that altering Type A behavior reduced the chances of a second attack by almost 40 percent.

The difficulty of diagnosing Type A behavior may explain some of these conflicting results. Researchers have yet to come up with objective ways of rating Type A components, and it's been argued that questionnaires miss unwritten cues and do not account reliably for differences in socioeconomic groups.

Some evidence suggests the constellation of behavior traits that adds up to Type A behavior may be too broad to pin down the cardiac connection. It's possible certain specific Type A components—hostility and anger—are the key contributors to heart disease, say Duke University internist Redford Williams and University of Maryland psychologist Theodore Dembroski.

Each of the many times a day Type A's get irritated and angry, their bodies convert to the alarm mode. The heart works extra hard, blood pressure goes up, and to counter the possibility of injury, the liver increases its output of cholesterol. With high cholesterol levels an established risk factor for heart disease, these hotheaded, easily angered people may become candidates for a heart attack.

Destructive, Type A anger is more likely to be triggered by small irritations and hassles—the little insults of everyday life—than rare crises such as job loss or divorce. In one job-stress study of policemen the men rated "excessive paperwork" almost as traumatic as physical attack. And in another study high-school teachers ranked paperwork second only to inadequate salary in stress severity. Day after day, the anger we waste on trivia, in traffic jams and ticket lines, and the "urge to kill" that boils up regularly are most likely to act upon the victims we least intend—ourselves.

Dissecting Type A behavior and its biological consequences is likely to keep researchers busy for some time. But if you feel yourself trapped in a web of daily indignities, if anger and rage flare with every new frustration, it may be time to take steps against a potentially lethal way of life. To give yourself a simple mental-stress checkup, you may wish to try the

Job-Stress Index on p.24 and the Temper Test below, developed by psychologist Charles L. Spielberger, a stress-management expert at the University of South Florida.

Temper Test

Dr. Spielberger has developed an anger test—the State-Trait Anger Scale (STAS)—that measures both the trait (general tendency to become angry) and the state (the intensity of angry feelings at a particular moment). High STAS scores have turned out to relate to hypertension, perhaps the single most important risk factor in heart attacks. The STAS compares your anger level with that of the average man or woman. You might like to score yourself on the trait section of this test.

Temper Test: Are You Stress-Prone?

DIRECTIONS:

A number of statements that people have used to describe themselves are given below. Read each statement and then circle the appropriate number to indicate how you *generally* feel. There are no right or wrong answers. Do not spend too much time on any one statement, but give the answer that seems to describe how you *generally* feel.

	Almost Never	Some-times	Often	Almost Always
1. I am quick-tempered	1	2	3	4
2. I have a fiery temper.	1	2	3	4
3. I am a hotheaded person.	1	2	3	4
4. I get angry when I'm slowed down by others' mistakes.	1	2	3	4
5. I feel annoyed when I am not given recognition for good work	1	2	3	4
6. I fly off the handle	1	2	3	4
7. When I get angry, I say nasty things	1	2	3	4
8. It makes me furious when I am criticized in front of others	1	2	3	4
9. When I get frustrated, I feel like hitting someone	1	2	3	4
10. I feel infuriated when I do a good job and get a poor evaluation	1	2	3	4

Total Points _____

Score Yourself: Counting the points (1 to 4) that you score on each item, add up the total and find where it places you in the percentile ranks. A man who scores 17, or a woman who scores 18, is just about average, at the 50th percentile.

A person who scores below 13 is down in the safe zones, perhaps unresponsive to situations that provoke others. A score of 23 or higher puts you up among the hotheads.

Percentile Ranks for Trait Anger

Percentile Ranks	Trait Anger Females	Males
95	28	28
85	23	23
75	21	21
50	18	17
25	15	14
15	14	13
5	12	11

Job-Stress Index: Are You Hassled?

DIRECTIONS:

This survey lists ten job-related events that have been identified as stressful by employees working in different settings. Read each item and circle the number that indicates the approximate number of times during the past month you have been upset or bothered by each event.

Number of Occurrences During Past Month

1. I have been bothered by fellow workers not doing their job	0	1	2	3+
2. I've had inadequate support from my supervisor	0	1	2	3+
3. I've had problems getting along with coworkers	0	1	2	3+
4. I've had trouble getting along with my supervisor	0	1	2	3+
5. I've felt pressed to make critical on-the-spot decisions	0	1	2	3+
6. I've been bothered that there aren't enough people to handle the job	0	1	2	3+
7. I've felt a lack of participation in policy decisions	0	1	2	3+
8. I've been concerned about my inadequate salary	0	1	2	3+
9. I've been troubled by a lack of recognition for good work	0	1	2	3+
10. I've been frustrated by excessive paperwork	0	1	2	3+

Total Points _____

Score Yourself: To determine how your stress compares with other workers, add up the points that you circled for each item (0-3). Your score will be between 0 and 30. If you score between 5 and 7, you are about average in how often you experience job-related stress. If you score higher than 9, you may have cause for concern. At 4 or lower, you have a relatively nonstressful job.

Double-Barreled Danger: 20+ and 9+
If you score higher than 20 on the temper test, and if your score is higher than 9 on the job-stress index, you've got a dangerous combination going. Better cool yourself or the job.

Double-digit job stress points to trouble, especially if your personality runs high in irritability and temper. Remember the double-barreled effect: If your personality makes you anger-prone, you have to watch out for jobs high in petty annoyances.

Job-Stress Index

Every job has its share of hassles and tensions. Dr. Spielberger's test (above) measures the level of stress in a job. It may give you a rough estimate of whether you and your job form a lethal combination.

COPING WITH STRESS

The tests you've just taken should provide some insight into how you deal with certain types of stress. But more important, you needn't be a bona fide Type A to benefit from stress-reduction techniques. In fact, behavior may fall on a continuum from the extremes of laid-back Type B behavior to classic Type A. At times, many of us feel life is whipping us on. A way of slowing the pace would certainly be welcome.

Sometimes just becoming aware of the source of hassles can make a difference. Improving time management, shifting priorities, and putting out small brushfires before the flames erupt are time-honored ways of taming job stress. There are also some basic behavior changes you can make that may ease you into a more relaxed lifestyle:

■ The most immediate stress antidote is to learn to relax. The method you choose is, of course, a matter of personal taste and individual stress style. But try to set aside twenty minutes a day for your overall relaxation "therapy," whether it's meditation, progressive relaxation, or noncompetitive exercise.

■ Be sensitive to how you think and react, particularly when you find yourself getting angry, irritable, or impatient. Learn to recognize negative "self-talk"—those inner monologues that arouse and anger you. When minor annoyances upset you, ask yourself, "What am I telling myself? What will this accomplish?"

■ Cultivate the *life*saving graces—the ability to find the humor in a situation or admit you're wrong. There's an inner strength, not weakness, in being able to admit you've made a mistake.

■ Slow down and try to be more patient. Take time to talk to people, to be friendly and neighborly. And when you do talk, try a more leisurely, less emphatic style. Gesture less abruptly with your head and hands and cut down on fidgeting and jiggling. Your conversational style, as we shall see in the next section, reverberates throughout your body, bringing about significant cardiovascular changes.

THE ART OF TALKING

From the first "da-da" to the final amen, we live our lives as talking animals. But for the most part, we talk without thinking about how conversation registers in our bodies. Whenever human beings communicate—even a pleasant chat about the weather or a grade-school recitation of the ABCs—heart rate increases and blood pressure rises. Dr. James J. Lynch, codirector of the Center for the Study of Human Psychophysiology at the University of Maryland Medical School, has spent years studying the physiology of communication and has described the work presented here in his book *The Language of the Heart.*

In a study of 178 people nine to eighty-three years old, 98 percent showed a blood-pressure increase while speaking, as expected. However, Lynch found the increase was much greater for hypertensives. In another study of thirty hypertensive patients, speech caused the blood pressure of sixteen to soar well into the danger zone. Though these patients often smiled and appeared outwardly calm, the researchers noticed that many of them tended to talk fast and loud, interrupt and speak over other people, and punctuate words with emphatic gestures. In fact, this kind of impulsive, impatient speech is a classic sign of Type A behavior.

To test the theory that style of speech may physically drive up blood pressure, thirty volunteers with normal pressure were asked to read aloud—first at their usual speed and then much more rapidly. At a normal pace average pressure rose from 118/65 to 125/70. "Speed reading" drove this up to 130/75. Lynch's experiment suggested that by learning to speak more slowly and breathing more regularly, hypertensives might be able to control pressure surges.

But breathlessness is only part of the story. Blood pressure is driven as much by the emotional implications of communicating as the physical act of talking. Deaf people using sign language responded the same way, whereas schizophrenics, who have extreme difficulty communicating with others, showed no change in blood pressure when they talked.

Talking, however, isn't all that counts, says Lynch. The simple act of conversing has a seesaw effect on blood pressure. The rise in pressure produced by speaking is balanced by a drop when we pause to listen. Ordinarily, this talk-listen combination keeps blood pressure evenly regulated.

But what if the listening side of the equation is missing? People with chronic hypertension not only may register an abnormal blood pressure surge while speaking, but they may also fail to listen when others speak. This deprives them of a natural way to lower pressure, says Lynch. Many of these people speak and listen defensively—a pattern they've often learned in childhood.

Lynch's research suggests that though most people lower their blood pressure during the listening phase of a conversation, hypertensives frequently don't use this natural way to relax. The importance of mastering the art of listening can be seen, says Lynch, in the "orienting reflex," which Pavlov discovered in the early 1900s. When a dog hears a soft sound or sees a sudden movement, Pavlov noted, it will stop everything and focus on the change. Later, other investigators discovered that as part of the response, the dog's heart rate slows.

Since Pavlov's time other scientists have found evidence of the orienting response in people. In one recent experiment, Dr. Aaron Katcher and his associate, Dr. Alan Beck, at the University of Pennsylvania charted people's blood pressure during three activities: reading out loud, staring at a blank wall, and watching fish swimming in a tank.

As expected, Katcher found that blood pressure was highest while speaking. But fish watching produced readings even lower than simply sitting and doing nothing. Whether watching fish in a tank or petting a dog or cat, paying calm attention to something outside yourself can trigger the orienting response and help bring blood pressure down. This may be one reason why teaching people to focus on something other than themselves—meditation and relaxation training—seems to be effective in lowering blood pressure.

Here are a few techniques to help modulate your blood pressure during conversation.

■ Slow your speech down. To make sure you breathe while you talk, imagine placing commas in your sentences. At every comma, take a breath.

■ Speak with your listeners in mind, and try to listen more than you speak.

■ Become aware of your body while you speak or are spoken to. Are you becoming tense, impatient? Are your fists clenched?

■ Try to become more a part of the world around you, whether that means getting a pet, growing plants, or even watching television if that makes you feel connected.

EXERCISE

We are becoming a nation of exercise nuts. We exercise for fitness and weight control; we exercise to keep our hearts healthy, by improving circulation and defusing stress. And we also exercise for sanity—fun and sheer joy. In Chapter 2 we prescribed vigorous exercise as a useful overall relaxer. Not only does it give stiff, tense muscles a good stretch, but exercise is a superb way of short-circuiting the endless erosive circling of worrisome thoughts. Move! Jump about for a while, and your mind must turn off. Afterward, those scattered thoughts

may not be able to reassemble so quickly.

But regular aerobic exercise appears to have another benefit. It may give your body an edge when sudden stress—a work deadline, a speech—sounds an alarm. Workouts may condition your body by providing a safer, less intense form of the physiological stress response—racing heart, increased blood pressure, and increased production of norepinephrine, a stress hormone related to adrenaline.

It is not clear how this works, but it's possible that exercise increases your body's reserves of norepinephrine, so it needs to produce less when you're in a sudden jam. Or workouts may enhance physiological efficiency so that less hormone is needed to mobilize the same amount of energy. Psychologist Richard Dienstbier of the University of Nebraska notes that athletes react more calmly in stressful situations than healthy but untrained people.

But go easy. Too much exercise can itself be stressful. Unlike moderate runs, marathons may impair your ability to cope with stress. And competitive thinking during briefer workouts may raise norepinephrine levels excessively. Instead, make workouts easier by concentrating on soothing thoughts. Psychologist Kenneth France at Shippensburg University in Pennsylvania found that when exercisers focused on competitive cues such as "push," "harder," "faster," they more than doubled their norepinephrine levels over days when they concentrated on gentle words, such as "steady" or "smooth."

Moderate aerobic exercise can also calm an anxious body by providing a positive channel for nervous energy. Even a single moderate "dose" of exercise can have a tranquilizing effect on muscle tension, says exercise psychologist Herbert de Vries.

And if you suspect you have Type A tendencies in your approach to challenge, exercise may help you unwind by providing "time out" and physical separation from work—but only if you turn off the stopwatch in your head. Don't take on exercise in an obsessive, goal-oriented way. But if you stick to a moderate, relaxed program, exercise can help Type A's get some Type B leverage in their lives.

The heart does indeed have its reasons. And we'd be wise to heed them. Your goal: Be alert to angry, driven behavior and try to cool it; slow down, listen, and laugh; finally, break the mental stress spiral with relaxation techniques and exercise.

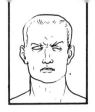

Part II: The Tension Trail
Chapter 4
Headache Healers

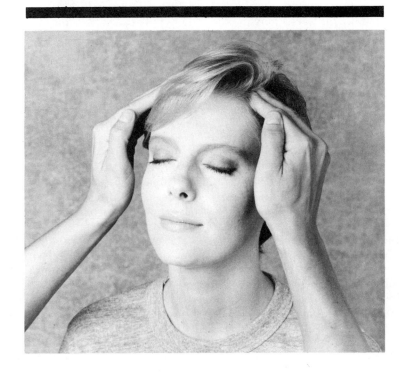

If crushing headaches regularly plow up your head, reducing your mind to mush, you may ask yourself: "Why me? Why now? Is it biochemistry? Personality? Stress? Will it help to relax and unwind?" If you knew the cause, you tell yourself, you could find an appropriate treatment.

Unfortunately, the experts can't always tell what's causing that pain in your skull. But they do know head pain generally signals a body at odds with itself. The more you know about the natural history of your headaches, the more you can do to bring your body into balance.

Even if doctors aren't certain about the origins of certain types of headache, they are becoming more sophisticated about treatment. They now know more about the best use of different headache remedies—drugs, relaxation techniques, and changes in diet. For example, some painkillers, even aspirin and acetaminophen, taken daily for weeks may make headaches worse, perhaps by overloading biochemical pain receptors in the brain. As for that old standby, aspirin, there's a simple rule of thumb: If two aspirins are going to help, they'll do it in twenty to thirty minutes. If the pain goes away in two minutes or in two hours, it's not the aspirin that's responsible.

There are four basic types of headache. *Tension* headaches, the most common, are caused by involuntary contractions of the scalp, head, and neck muscles. Tension headaches, not surprisingly, are best treated with relaxation therapy and are the main form of head misery this book hopes to soothe away.

The other types include *vascular* headaches, caused by swollen blood vessels that irritate nearby pain receptors. Migraine, cluster (a severe form of migraine), hangover, hunger, "ice-cream," and menstrual headaches are all vascular in origin. *Secondary* headaches, caused by disease or head injury, require prompt treatment but are rare—less than 2 percent of all headaches. *Psychological* or "conversion" headaches are triggered by emotional stress and are entirely mental in origin. The pain is real, but no muscles or blood vessels are involved.

Many headaches—particularly the common tension variety—can be eased without expensive tests, prescription drugs, or long-term professional treatment. The first step in soothing the throbbing pain is quick self-diagnosis. The flowchart on p. 30–31 will help you determine the type of headache you have and what sets it off.

WHO GETS HEADACHES

Few headaches are either "all in the mind" or "merely physical"; the majority fall somewhere in between. A combination of heredity, constitution, and personality determines who will be most susceptible.

For example, the throbbing pain of a migraine begins when scalp blood vessels shrink and swell; chemicals leak through the vessel walls, inflame nearby tissues, and stimulate nerve endings to send pain signals to the brain. Migraine victims seem to inherit bodies and biochemistries that are unusually vulnerable; they are born with a blood-vessel system that is easily dilated. But emotional stress—as well as changes in air pressure, odors, and other signals—may be triggers that throw the system out of whack.

Surveys of college women show that the hard-driving Type A behavior pattern increases the risk of both migraine and tension headaches. But despite such clues, the stereotype of the neurotic, high-strung headache sufferer doesn't always hold.

Factors other than personality—such as age and sex—do affect headache risk. Women, for example, seek medical care for headaches more often than men. But that doesn't prove they actually get more headaches; they may just feel more comfortable complaining about them. And both sexes are more prone to headaches between the ages of thirty and sixty.

Children were once thought to be almost immune, but new research shows that's not true. Dr. David Rothner, chief of pediatric neurology at the Cleveland Clinic Foundation, estimates that one fifth of American youngsters have migraine or serious tension headaches, and that 40 percent of all migraine sufferers have their first bout before they are fifteen.

WHAT TRIGGERS YOUR PAIN?

To prevent headaches, first find the fuse that sets them off. Take a careful history, noting the dates and times of attacks, along with the physical, mental, and emotional activities of your day. You may find certain foods, weather changes, light, or kinds of stress or illness are your triggers.

Does the headache develop immediately after exercise? In the morning when you wake up? Only on weekends? Notice whether you clench your teeth (see Chapter 5, "Jawbones," p. 39), how you read a book, and whether lighting and seating at work cause strain (see Chapter 14, "Pain in the Office," p.159). Write down any medicines you take and how often. Is there a headache-linked pattern? Tracking these variables may help you pin down the cause of your headache.

If your headaches started recently, think about changes in diet, furnishings, general health, and location. When a native New Englander experienced dull, throbbing pain around the scalp and neck on a golf vacation in Arizona, he traced it to the intensity of the light on the desert courses. Sunglasses eliminated his muscle-tension headaches, caused by squinting against the glare.

The environment often affects headaches. Migraines are more common when the barometer rises or falls dramatically, less common in cloudy, rainy weather. Air pollution can also be a migraine trigger.

Diet is a factor in 15 to 20 percent of all headache patients, estimates Dr. Seymour Diamond, director of Chicago's Diamond Headache Clinic. Though doctors are still debating whether "dietary migraine" exists, there's a growing consensus that some foods can be painful for some people. The most troublesome substances seem to be chocolate, alcohol, hard cheese, nuts, and citrus fruits, as well as preservatives and taste enhancers such as monosodium glutamate (MSG) and nitrates.

A word of caution: If your headaches suddenly become more intense or frequent, check with your doctor. Be especially cautious if the pains come with blurred vision, nausea, numbness, tingling in arms or legs, strange or strong odors no one else detects, sweating, or flushing.

Once you understand your headache, you have a much better chance of treating it. "With the right diagnosis, more than 90 percent of headache sufferers will improve the quality of their lives. Instead of headaches managing people, people are managing their headaches," says Dr. William Speed, a headache consultant at the Johns Hopkins Pain Treatment Center.

MIGRAINE

If migraine is the cause, biofeedback, relaxation, and medication may be in order. You may be able to short-circuit attacks by recognizing the signs that one is about to begin and, using a relaxer at that point, head off the painful second phase. During the first phase, before pain begins, some people get specific signals the headache is starting. For some the sign is nausea, for others a hypersensitivity to light and sound. Still others experience a distinctive visual pattern, like cracked glass floating in the visual field.

If you know your signs and have practiced a relaxer such as meditation or muscle relaxation, you may be one of the lucky people who can use this cue to start relaxation therapy. This can reverse blood-flow patterns and avert the painful second phase of the migraine.

But don't wait for the headache to take over your head. It's important to practice your soothing routines regularly so that your relaxing reflexes are sufficiently developed to come to your rescue quickly and automatically when a headache is lurking in the wings. If you get migraines regularly, you know it is worth a try.

WHEN TENSION IS THE PROBLEM

If tension headaches are shutting you down, the simple regimens provided here will help loosen tense muscles, break the tension spiral, and give you drug-free relief. Again, your best bet for avoiding or ending headaches is to have a "relaxercise" you do every day. In general, you'll be less likely to set off the muscle-tension spiral and you'll be buffered against routine stresses and hassles. Some people find daily progressive relaxation (whole-body deep relaxation) helpful. More specifically, if you are on the fringe of a headache, you may prevent full-blown agony by doing your relaxer right then and there.

If that doesn't work, and aspirin and acetaminophen don't appeal to you, here are some other remedies you can try.

Start here.

If the answer to any
question in a box is
"Yes," follow that arrow;
otherwise, follow the "No"
arrow.
Are your headaches chronic
or recurrent?

Signs of Something More Serious
Numbness, blurred vision, fever, balance problems, light sensitivity, convulsions, disorientation and memory loss in conjunction with headaches are all warning signals. You should see a physician if you experience any of them.

NO ▼
Are you older than 45? Have you recently lost weight, experienced pain in hips or shoulders? Do you have throbbing temple headaches you never had before that are worse at night? Do you have blind spots or blurred vision? Do the blood vessels you can see at your temple feel tender or swollen?

YES ▼
Is there any evidence of diseases of your eyes, nose, sinuses? Have you had a head injury? Do you suffer from food allergies? Are you sensitive to cold or to drugs such as steroids? Do you have high blood pressure or blood sugar disorder? Do you have back or neck problems of long standing?

NO

YES ← You probably have **temporal arthritis,** which requires treatment by a physician.

NO

You may have any of the following: If you have a "headband" pressure type of ache that is most severe in the morning, you may have **high blood pressure** headache. Treatment: drugs and diet to control high blood pressure.

If there is pain, swelling and tenderness over the forehead, nose or cheek, you may have **sinus** headache. Treatment: moist heat, painkillers, medication to drain sinuses and to treat inflammation and infection.

If pain is accompanied by congestion in nose and watery eyes, you probably have an **allergy** headache. Treatment: antihistamines and allergy shots.

YES ← Are you having symptoms of ear or sinus infection, dental problems? Do you have high blood pressure? Are you taking drugs that produce any side effects?

NO

YES ← You probably have **secondary inflammatory headache.** Treatment: Try simple home remedies for a few days. If symptoms persist, see your physician.

Have you now, or have you recently had a serious infection, viral illness such as flu?

NO

Are you under 30? **YES**   **NO**

Are your headaches mostly on one side of your head, **YES** periodic, throbbing, accompanied by nausea? Are there close relatives with these kinds of headache? **NO**

Chart Your Pain Away

Does your pain focus around one eye? Do you have spasms or cascades of pain accompanied by red eyes and nasal congestion? Is the pain excruciating? Are you male and between 20 and 30?

NO | **YES**

Does your headache feel like a band of pressure on both sides of your head? Are your headaches frequent or constant? Are you depressed or anxious?

NO | **YES**

Consult your doctor. Consider a good checkup for anemia, kidney problems, hardening of the arteries, heart disease, serious depression, glaucoma, arthritis.

If there is still no apparent cause, relax, try simple home remedies such as nonprescription pain-relievers, ice packs, rest. Be alert to changing patterns, but your headache is probably not very serious.

You probably have **common migraine**. Treatment: painkillers, ice packs, rest, medications that constrict blood vessels (ergotamine products), anti-nausea drugs, beta blockers, anti-prostaglandins, biofeedback.

NO ↑

Do you have visual "auras," other sensory signals such as perception of unusual odors, or other physical symptoms 30 minutes before the pain begins?

YES →

You probably have **cluster** headache or **neuralgia.** Treatment: ergotamine products, oxygen inhalation and occasionally nerve surgery. Alcohol, heavy smoking, fatigue and stress may all be triggers.

You probably have **muscle tension** headache, the most common of all headaches. Treatment: relaxation, sleep, nonprescription pain relievers, ice, antispasmodics, antidepressants, psychotherapy, biofeedback. Try to avoid physical or emotional stress triggers. If pain is around temple and forehead, it may be simple **eyestrain**.

You probably have **classic migraine**. Treatment: biofeedback, relaxation and vasoconstrictors such as ergotamine will abort pain during aura phase before pain begins. Once pain has begun, treatment is same as for common migraine.

NO ↑

Do these signals persist after the headache or during it?

YES ↓

You probably have a complicated form of migraine that requires professional diagnosis.

Some other headaches are due to obvious causes and their diagnosis will be less ambiguous.
Menstrual headache: pain that occurs before, during or just after menstruation, or at mid-cycle. Treatment: same as migraine.
Ice-cream headache: pain in forehead, nose or ears that occurs suddenly after eating or drinking cold foods. Treatment: Eat cold foods in small portions and allow them to warm slightly in front of mouth.
Hangover headache: throbbing head pain following the consumption of alcoholic beverages. Treatment: Drink nonalcoholic beverages, especially fruit juices.
Temporomandibular joint syndrome (TMJ): jaw pain that occurs suddenly, often while chewing or yawning. Treatment: Consult a dentist

31

Quick Rub

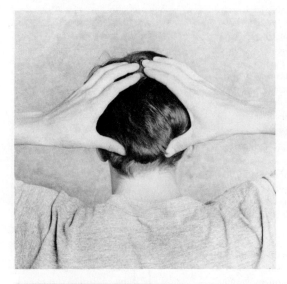 Put your fingers on your head, with your thumbs at the back, on the base of the skull. Gently massage around the base from the ears to the center, and back again. Do it slowly, four or five times—or longer if you want.

Unknotting the Trapezius

Have your shoulders climbed up around your ears? You may be shrugging yourself into a trapezius-triggered headache. A heating pad, hot bath, or shower can help by warming knotted neck and shoulder muscles, increasing blood flow and oxygen supply. Beginning on p. 65, in Chapter 7, "Necksavers," you'll find a selection of moves aimed at detensing an uptight trapezius.

Jammed Jaw

For some people headache pain may be traced to a clenched jaw or teeth grinding, a condition known as bruxism. If your mouth is closed so tightly your teeth touch, you may be holding tension in your jaw without realizing it. To relieve a headache due to jaw tension, find the spot below and in front of your ears— the masseter—that bulges out when you clench your jaw. Now let your jaw drop open as you massage that area with your fingertips in a light, circular motion. If an ailing jaw is a serious problem, turn to the next chapter, "Jawbones," p.39, for a first-aid kit.

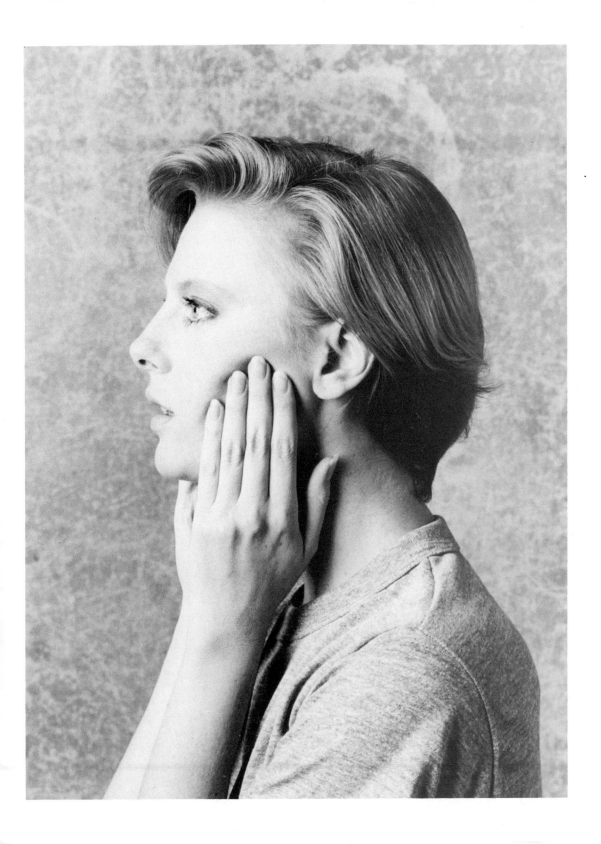

Scalped

The scalp is more than a planting ground for hair. There are muscles throughout this section of skin, though we rarely notice them. Yet many tension headaches are caused by constriction of the blood vessels that feed these muscles. You'll find these special scalp treats a first-rate investment if your head is "scalping" you.

The Hair Pull

This one's simple. Grab a hunk of hair with each hand. Gently tug, bobbing your hand slightly for a few seconds. Then grab another hunk and do the same, moving on through your entire head of hair.

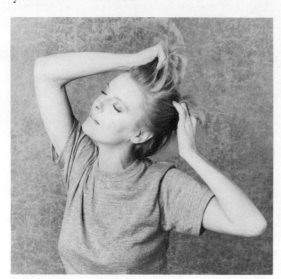

Scalp-plus Massage

This massage focuses on the main tension headache culprits—jaw, forehead, temple, base of the skull, and, of course, scalp.

Place both hands on top of your head, so they meet in the midline. Using all fingers of both hands, press and massage hard in circular movements, covering the entire scalp from forehead to nape of the neck, from ear to ear. Pay particular attention—use your thumbs—to the point where the base of the skull meets the neck.

With your fingers, massage your temples in a firm, circular motion for a minute or so. Then slowly massage your way across your forehead until your hands meet in the middle. Move back to the temples again.

Now bring your hands down on either side to the point just in front of the earlobes where you feel a bulge when you clench your jaw. Massage there, as you did your temples.

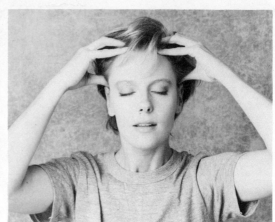

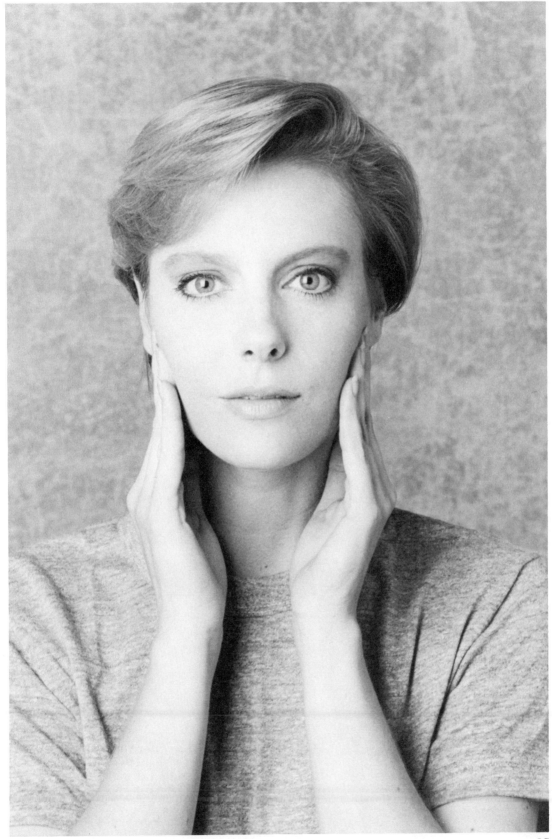

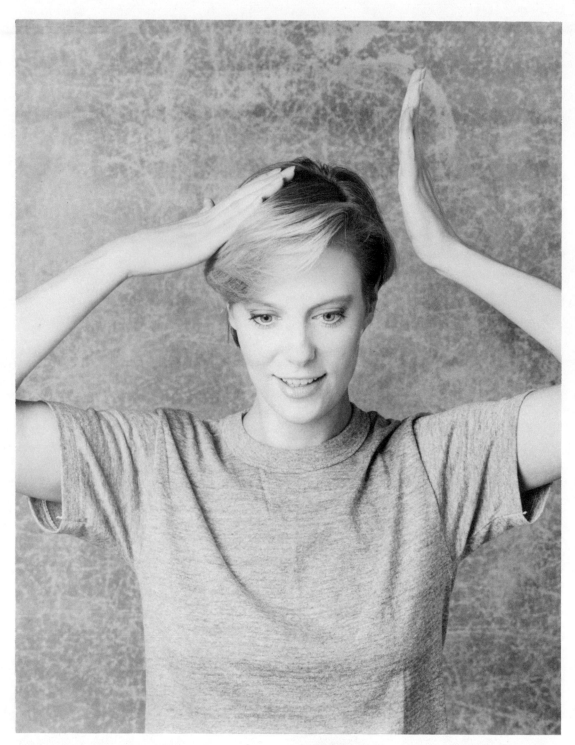

The Slap

Here's a good one for the shower on those mornings when it's hard to wake up. With your hand open, rapidly pat and slap your scalp. Make several circuits; be brisk but light. For an extra stimulating treat, keep going on down the arms, chest, legs—anywhere you can reach.

Massage: With a Partner—and Without

Several simple massages have been found to help, even banish, muscle-tension headaches. They are worth a try. Though these include a partner, experiment a bit. You may be able to manage most of the moves yourself.

Forehead Strokes
Facing your partner, put your thumbs together at your partner's hairline, in the midline of the forehead. Your fingers should spread out to the sides. Squeezing lightly, stroke the forehead, moving your thumbs out to the sides. Stroke just firmly enough so that the forehead skin stretches. Then return your hands to the original position and repeat several times.

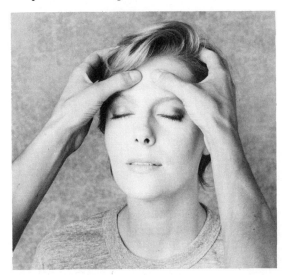

Sinus Rub
Try this one for a sinus headache. Use a stroke similar to the one above, starting with your thumbs at the tip of the person's nose, your fingers bunched at the temples. Now rub up toward the nose. As your thumbs reach the hollow between the eyes and nose, use them to make deep strokes over the eyebrows, out toward the temples. Then slide back to the starting position and repeat several times.

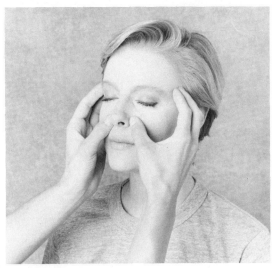

Temples
Put your fingertips in the skull sockets at the temples. Rub in a spiraling circle around the temples, expanding out to the hairline, then spiraling back again.

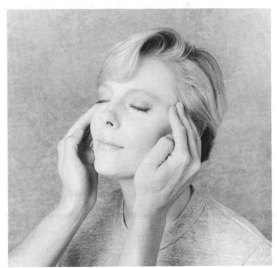

Scalp

Constricted scalp muscles are responsible for many a tension headache. A scalp massage is a good way to deal with this kind of headache.

Start with your fingertips just above the hairline, and work up slowly into the headache-sufferer's hair. Move down toward the front of the ear, then back over the ear into the hair, in a circle around the ear to the base of the skull.

Repeat this move several times, each time moving higher onto the head, ending at a different point at the base of the skull—always going toward the center of the neck. Finally, you will have covered most of the scalp.

Base of Head

The muscles at the back of the skull often contribute to headaches. With your fingertips, work along the base of the skull in firm, circular movements, from the bumps behind the ears at the base of the head, along the bottom of the skull, to the center. Now go back again.

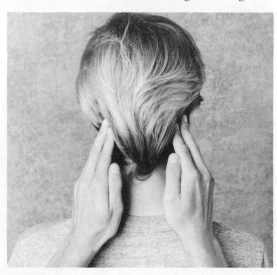

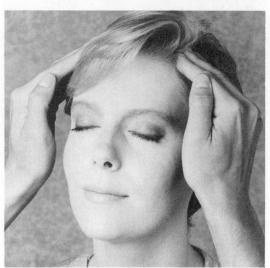

Shoulders

As mentioned above, a good trapezius massage can do wonders for some headaches. See Chapter 7, "Necksavers," p.63, for shoulder massages.

Our headache package ends with a reminder to prepare your defenses ahead of time, particularly if muscle tension is the source of your woes. A spot scan—head, neck, and shoulders—plus progressive relaxation or meditation as overall relaxers may drive off gathering headache demons. But to head off that headache, practice now.

Chapter 5

Jawbones:
TMJ
Syndrome

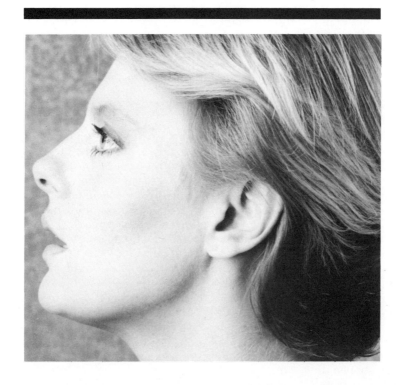

The pressure's on! Grit your teeth, clench your jaw—hang on and hang in. Think about it, though. Jaw clenching has nothing to do with overcoming obstacles and dealing with stress. Yet because the jaw is part of the emotionally expressive musculature of the face, we may automatically funnel stress into this hard-working joint.

Gritting, grinding, or clenching may become a habit, expressing a free-floating level of anxiety that surfaces even at night. The result, in many cases, is TMJ syndrome—pain or dysfunction of the temporomandibular joint, the hinge that joins the jaw to the skull. Because the cause of TMJ problems may be difficult to diagnose, it's useful to understand the debate about what makes this joint act up.

A once-obscure joint disorder, known to Hippocrates, TMJ disorder has recently achieved the status of "disease of the year." This so-called menace is alleged to afflict some 47 million Americans. However many it really affects, it's useful to know what to do—and not do—about it if your jaw is acting up.

A complex of bone, cartilage, nerve, and muscle, the TMJ is as vulnerable as any joint to injury or arthritis. But its special duties—moving the lower jaw open and shut for talking and eating—create special hazards. The joint bears the enormous forces of chewing and absorbs the shock waves from nervous gritting or grinding (bruxism) of the teeth.

The joint's inner cartilage disk can wear and tear, and tension and spasm can grip the muscles that move the joint. The heavily exercised main chewing muscles—the masseter and temporalis—are the most susceptible to tension. Finally, unlike any other joint, the TMJ's action is also governed by outside forces: the condition and position of the teeth.

No one disputes the fact that a malfunctioning TMJ can produce pain, particularly along the jaw or in the area of the ear or neck. There

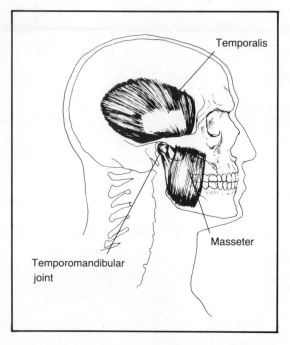

may be difficulty eating and talking, a clicking or popping sound may be heard when the mouth opens or closes, or the jaw may even lock into one position. Some tension headaches can be traced to an unhappy TMJ.

Why does the joint misbehave? There are three possible causes, each with its own backers: emotional stress, mechanical pressure, and bad bite. Nine out of ten people with an ailing TMJ have tight jaw muscles, resulting from stress-related muscle tension, says oral surgeon Daniel L. Laskin, director of the TMJ and Facial Pain Center at the Medical College of Virginia. Years of using the mouth to absorb stress—jutting the jaw or clenching or grinding teeth—tightens the jaw muscles around the joint.

Others say the main trouble is malocclusion of the teeth, with or without muscle tension. Poor alignment of the teeth and jaw, perhaps developing over the years, impedes the natural movement of the TMJ, so that it takes a battering every time the mouth opens and shuts.

What to do about the problem is a matter of wide controversy, affecting the mouths—and pocketbooks—of millions of Americans. A safe, conservative approach is to try muscle-relaxation therapy.

HEALTH MENACE?

Despite this simple prescription, there are those who perceive the jaw hinge as a serious health hazard. They accuse it of sapping athletic prowess and afflicting ordinary mortals with everything from toothaches and backaches to hemorrhoids, scoliosis, and even schizophrenia. TMJ clinics have sprung up around the country, and some oral surgeons are even breaking jaws, theorizing that changing the bite will ease the pain.

All this may mean that a long-neglected health problem is finally getting overdue attention. But the hard evidence indicates TMJ disorder is "overdiagnosed and overtreated," says Dr. Laskin. "It's become a cult," agrees Dr. David Keith, assistant professor of oral and maxillofacial surgery at Harvard Dental School.

Part of the problem, according to a number of observers, is that orthopedists have left it to the dentists, spurning it for more glamorous joints—shoulder, hip, knee, ankle. But until recently, dentists were busy filling cavities. Now fluoride has changed dental practice, and some dentists have climbed on the TMJ bandwagon. There are books on how to double your dental practice with TMJ therapy, says Laskin.

The dentists' remedies include fitting customized biteplates ($200 to $2,000) to take the stress off the TMJ, or redesigning the dental landscape—building teeth up with caps, filing others down. Yet a conference convened by the American Dental Association in 1983 could find little scientific support for any single approach to TMJ—assuming therapy was necessary in the first place. The National Institute of Dental Research is now developing standards for diagnosing TMJ syndrome.

In addition, a clicking jaw need not signal TMJ dysfunction. Dr. Laskin notes that people with no pain or discomfort may make the same clicking, crunching, and gravelly sounds as those with a true TMJ problem. Harvard's Dr. Keith says 30 to 35 percent of healthy people have noisy joints, though no one knows whether such sounds presage TMJ trouble.

Despite the enormous number of people who believe they have a TMJ disorder, the American Dental Association has no idea how many need treatment. Only three of every ten patients claiming TMJ problems actually have them, says orthodontist Lawrence Harte, director of the New Jersey Center for Cranial Facial Pain in Livingston. "According to some dentists, everyone with pain in the jaw or head

has TMJ dysfunction," notes Dr. Seymour Diamond, head of Chicago's Diamond Headache Clinic. Of the forty new migraine patients he sees weekly, "three or four have had treatment for TMJ. In most cases, it's totally unwarranted," he says. However, Dr. Diamond and other headache experts do agree that some tension headaches may be triggered by a TMJ problem; relaxing the appropriate jaw muscles may ease this type of headache.

Until standards of TMJ diagnosis and treatment are established, it's up to people to protect themselves from needlessly expensive treatment. The best way, says Dr. Steven M. Goldman of Walnut Creek, California, past president of the American Academy of Craniomandibular Disorders, is to consult a knowledgeable dentist or one affiliated with a dental or medical school. Most of all, beware of any diagnosis of TMJ syndrome accompanied by a recommendation for extensive treatment without at least a lengthy interview with the doctor. Your dentist might also want a report from a neurologist or orthopedist, to rule out such problems as a tumor or bursitis.

Harvard's Dr. Keith advises: If there's no pain at the joint itself, there's probably no significant TMJ problem, even if you hear an occasional click when chewing. "If you feel fine, don't rush into treatment."

In a study Dr. Laskin conducted, 90 percent of TMJ patients got better whether given simple muscle-relaxation therapy or ambitious bite reconstruction. "Why use invasive, expensive treatment when simple therapies accomplish the same thing?" he asks. Dentists at the University of Tennessee Dental School in Memphis, for example, simply refer TMJ patients to physical therapists who help them break bad postural habits, such as head tilting while reading or talking.

SIMPLE SOOTHERS

So if you really have a balky jaw joint, here are some techniques that will help relax tense muscles and get your jaw back in working order. Jaw tension is actually a matter of degree; at its worst it becomes the agony of TMJ, but there are milder levels of jaw tension you may wish to ease.

There's a simple rule of thumb for assessing jaw tension: Your teeth should not be in contact except when swallowing or chewing. At other times there should be a slight separation between upper and lower levels. If not, you are holding tension in your jaw.

Jaw Awareness

Clenching your teeth is a habit you've learned; it can be unlearned. One simple solution is to cultivate the opposing habit—a slack jaw.

Let your mouth hang open, your jaw loose. That's a slack jaw, but it looks a bit foolish. So gently close your mouth, your lips together, but keep your jaw relaxed. Your top and bottom teeth should not meet when you close your mouth.

Remember the distinctive feeling of a relaxed jaw and try to return to it throughout the day. Tune in to your jaw from time to time to see how tense it is. Now relax—drop your jaw a bit and part your lips slightly.

It may be useful to find a reminder that will be a cue to check your jaw through the day—something you do regularly, like sit down or look at your watch. Each time, check your jaw and let it relax.

Jaw Drop. The quickest relaxer is simply to let your jaw drop, so that your mouth opens slightly. Now take a deep breath through your mouth and exhale with slight forcefulness, so that you can hear a "haaah." Repeat for five or six deep breaths, keeping your attention on your jaw. Let it drop open a bit more—at least mentally—with each exhalation.

Habits

Some "cures" are amazingly simple—give up chewing gum or switch telephone ears. If you spend hours on the phone, especially if you lean on a shoulder cradle, you may be putting too much pressure on your jaw.

Jaw Easers

Here's a set of relaxers designed to relieve pressure buildup in the jaw and the major connecting muscles.

■ Clasp your hands behind your neck (opposite), then with a firm movement, bring your elbows together in front of you. Slide your fingers apart, continuing the movement, and slide your hands forward along the sides of your head, your fingers pressing as they slide by your jawline to your chin. Do it three times. This is an odd exercise, but the firm, rhythmic movement helps release jaw tension.

■ Put each hand along your jaw on either side, heel of the hand at your chin, fingers pointing toward the ear. Gently push into the side of your jaw with your hands at the base of the ears. You should feel the jaw move slightly into the skull. Hold the press for a few moments. Repeat three times.

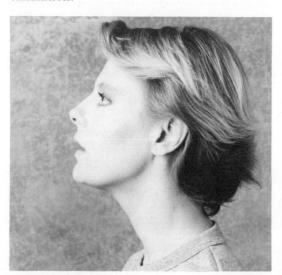

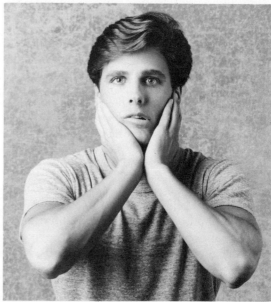

■ With your lips slightly parted and your jaw relaxed, use your fingertips to massage around the joint where jaw meets skull, just in front of the ears. Be firm. This simple jaw easer can be done any time you think of it during the day.

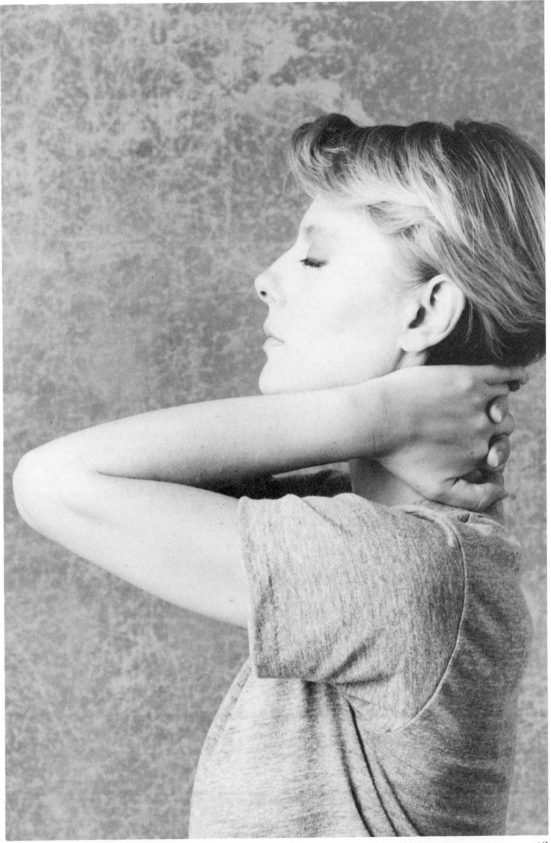

Jaw Stretches

Big Stretch

Nothing's simpler. Just opening your mouth as wide as possible gives your jaw muscles a good stretch. Try opening your mouth in the biggest O you can, stretching your lips in a circle. Hold it about fifteen seconds, then let your mouth close, keeping your jaw slack. Do this five or six times at several points during the day.

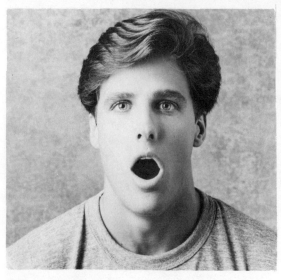

The Cork

A clenched jaw is a tense jaw. Clenching limits the jaw muscle's range of movement. The antidote is to hold the mouth open in a simple stretch that gradually lengthens the jaw muscles. Use a thermos bottle cork for this one (wine corks are too long). Ideally, assemble a variety of lengths, from about 1 inch to 1¾ inches.

Start with a cork you can place vertically between your teeth, while still able to open your mouth comfortably another quarter inch. If it's uncomfortable, switch to a shorter cork. You may drool a bit, so keep a tissue handy. And remember to breathe normally.

Once the cork is right, all you do is hold it between your teeth for a minute or two, longer if you wish. Gradually work up to longer corks and more time. If this muscle stretcher becomes part of your regular routine, try it while reading or doing something that doesn't require you to talk.

The Hinge

A good way to protect the jaw joint is to enlarge its range of movement and enhance awareness of the difference between the upper and lower jaw. Try this:

1. Think of your upper jaw as your skull and your lower jaw as a hinge that swings down from the base of the skull.

2. Hold your chin firmly between your thumb and fingers, and look straight ahead. Now open your mouth, not by lowering your chin, but by moving your entire skull upward. Your chin remains in its original position, and your head tilts back so that you are looking up at the ceiling.

3. Now close your mouth by bringing your lower lip up to meet the upper lip. At the end of the movement your head should stay tilted back. Starting from the new position, repeat the movement so your head tilts even more.

4. Reverse the motion. Starting with your head tipped back, drop your lower jaw; hold it in that position while you bring your upper jaw down to meet the lower—moving your entire head. Repeat once more until you are back at the starting position.

In sum, if a jammed jaw joint has been properly diagnosed as the cause of pain, chewing problems, or headaches, you may wish to pursue an expanded relaxation program or read still further. Suggested Reading, p. 189, lists a useful book by Dr. Harold Gelb. Above all, consult a knowledgeable doctor before heeding anyone who says your mouth needs redesigning.

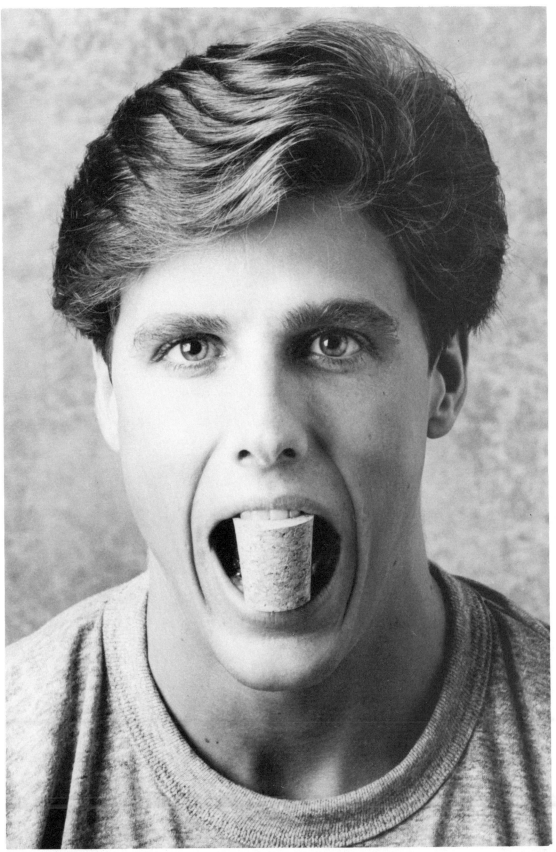

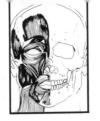

Chapter 6

Facesavers

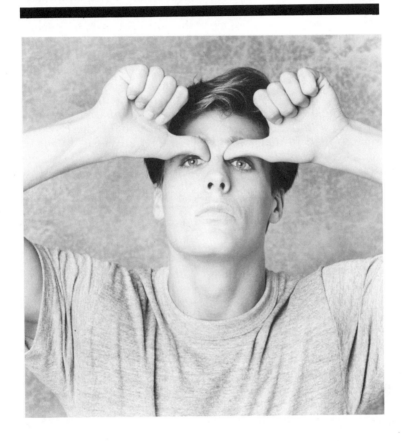

Of all the parts of your body, your face is unique: The world knows your face—it is you—and yet, unlike hips or hands, you can never really see it. Over one hundred muscles, exquisitely tuned to each nuance of feeling, to every fleeting mood, spend the waking day mirroring your emotions—or hiding your true feelings. Either way, the facial muscles get quite a workout, tensing and relaxing in (or out of) tune with your feelings.

When we are happy, surprised, or enthusiastic, face muscles make the matching maneuvers. If we are harried, worried, or depressed, sensitive muscles dutifully record a corresponding pattern of tension. Because the face muscles are so directly tied to our emotions, pressure and stress create a special burden.

Feeling worried and sad is a case in point. In a landmark study at Harvard, researchers found that patients who were depressed had chronically tensed corrugator muscles—the muscles that knit the brow into a frown. The patients had become so used to that level of tension, they weren't even aware their frown muscles were tense. Often, there was no visible sign of facial tension.

In a study on anxiety at Rutgers University, patients became less stressed when taught, through biofeedback, to relax their forehead muscles. As a result of such studies, teaching people to ease depression and anxiety by relaxing key facial muscles—specifically those that reflect negative emotions—has become a standard clinical tool.

Not surprisingly, in biofeedback training the face muscles are often used to gauge the level of tension throughout the body. A high general level of muscle tension will show up in the face; conversely, when the body relaxes, so does the face. But you don't need a biofeedback machine to relax your face. Instead, try these stretches, massages, facials, and other face treats.

STRETCHES

Despite the incredible work the facial muscles do during the day, many never get put through their full range of movement, and others stall in a fixed range of tension. A thorough workout can break these muscles out of their habitual patterns and leave them—and you—feeling awakened and relaxed. These exercises increase circulation and smooth away tension. During these stretches you'll look pretty strange, but by the end you should feel great.

Whether facial exercises cause wrinkles is the subject of an endless debate, since it's difficult to evaluate these effects on the human hide. Most cosmetic experts say pulling and stretching are bad for the skin; some draw the line at excessive stretching. Others, including many dermatologists, maintain that wrinkles are mainly a matter of genes and exposure to elements. So far, there's no answer; do what's best for your needs. In any case, there's little danger the few facial stretches recommended here will pose a wrinkle threat: Their main effect is on the muscles beneath the skin.

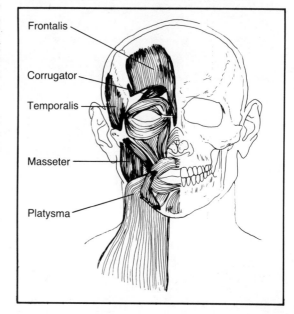

Frontalis

Corrugator

Temporalis

Masseter

Platysma

Chin and Mouth

The chin is sheathed by the largest muscle of the face, the platysma, which extends from the cheeks, jaws, and mouth down the neck to the chest. This muscle raises and lowers the chin, and controls that movement essential to every pouting child, pulling down the corners of the mouth.

Chin Workout

Draw down the corners of your mouth as though grimacing. Hold for six seconds.

With your lips together and without moving your head, twist your lips around in each direction: toward the left, the right, the bottom, the top. Do six full sequences of twists in each direction, for about a second each.

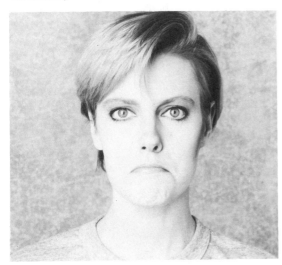

Lips

Purse your lips into an O as though you were going to whistle. Hold for six seconds.

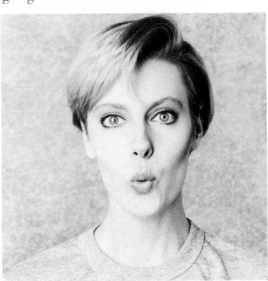

Mouth Stretch

Now stretch your mouth in the most open and wide smile you can, pulling your lips out to the side as far as they'll go. The weird result will give the muscles around your lips a stretch they rarely enjoy. Hold six seconds.

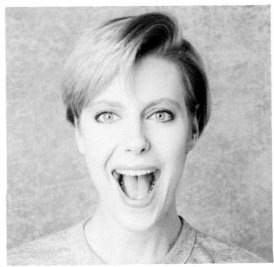

49

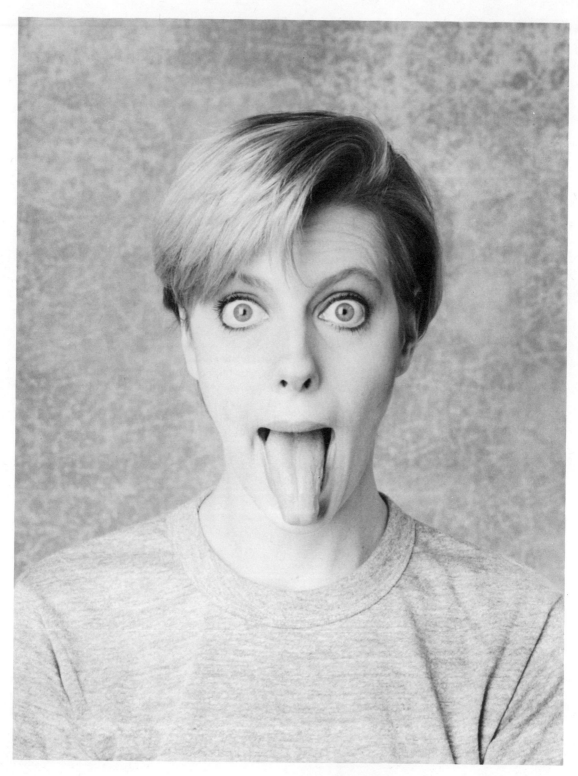

Yoga Lion Pose
Keep your back straight, open your mouth
wide, and stick your tongue as far out and
down as you can reach. As you do this, bug
your eyes wide open. Now, like a lion, inhale
deeply and exhale with a breathy "haaah!"

Eye Walks

The muscles that move the eyes do a great job of fine-tuning the gaze, but they rarely get a full workout. Here's a quick treat for them.

Imagine you're gazing at a huge clockface straight ahead of you. Keep your head erect and still as you swing your gaze in the widest arc, sweeping the clockface like a second hand, from 1 o'clock to 12 o'clock. See where the different hours are marked?

Now without moving your head, use your eye muscles to focus on 12 o'clock, then down to 6. Now head around the clock in the same pattern: 1-7, 2-8, 3-9, and so on back to 12. Repeat counterclockwise: 11-5, 10-4, 9-3, etc.

Eye Squeeze and Whole-Face Stretch

Keeping your head still and your gaze straight ahead, raise and lower your eyebrows as far as you can. Repeat eight to ten times in each direction, holding for a moment or two at the top and bottom. It might help to look in the mirror to be sure you move your eyebrows, not your head.

Next, switch to opening and closing your eyes in sequence. Widen your eyes, bugging them out. Raise your eyebrows and let your jaw drop open.

Then squeeze your eyes closed tight, letting your whole face scrunch up as part of the movement. Alternate opening and closing about ten times each. Vary the pace . . . quickly . . . slowly.

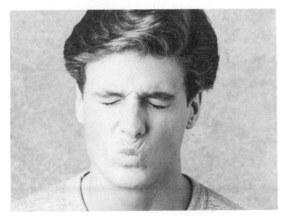

Now open and close your mouth. Open your mouth as wide as you can, so that you feel the muscles around your mouth and cheeks stretch fully.

Then screw up your mouth and wrinkle your nose while you squinch your eyes shut. Alter-

nate opening and squinching at varied paces for another cycle of six repetitions.

Now, finally, let your face rest, expressionless, your lips slightly parted, your jaw at ease, your brow smooth, your whole face relaxed.

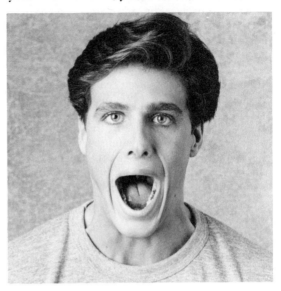

Free-form Stretches: Face Fun

To keep your face from getting too set in its ways, play with it from time to time. Look in a mirror and make faces. Snarl, show your teeth, let out a sound. Stick out your tongue. Give a Bronx cheer. Wrinkle your nose. Raise and lower your eyebrows. Pout, yawn, grimace. Scrunch up and open wide. Growl, laugh. Chew up a carrot or an apple.

Jaw Relaxers

Of all the face muscles, those that operate the jaw are the strongest. Because the main chewing muscle—the masseter—constantly works against resistance—food—it gets the most exercise. Yet for all this, the jaw is also particularly vulnerable to the ravages of tension. The masseter and the temporalis, the major chewing muscles, often react to tension by clenching the jaw tightly shut. Or the entire jaw complex may store tension, which causes other kinds of problems, from headaches to tooth grinding and jaw clenching (bruxism). If you're plagued by jaw problems, turn back to Chapter 5, "Jawbones," p.39, for a complete rescue kit.

 Jaw Drop. Here's a simple fix you've tried before. Let your jaw drop so that your mouth opens slightly. Breathe deeply through your mouth and exhale with slight forcefulness, so you can hear a "haaah." Repeat for five or six deep breaths, keeping your attention on your jaw. Let it drop open a bit more—at least mentally—each time you exhale.

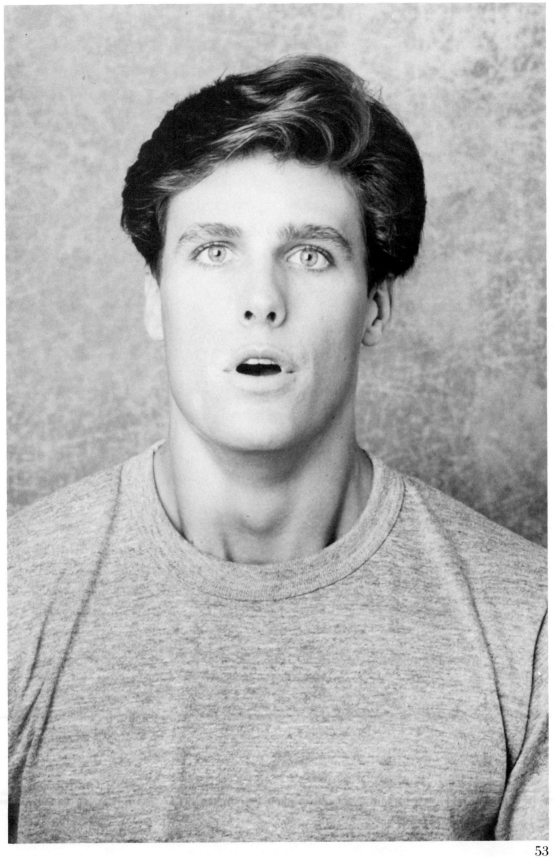

DO-IT-YOURSELF FACIAL MASSAGE

Face Rubs

A face rub is a quick way to bring more blood to your face. Start by putting your palms on your cheeks. Rub up and down briskly. It should take just a few moments before you feel your cheeks warming. Then move up to rub your temples and forehead, keeping up a brisk stroke. Then move down on either side of the bridge of your nose, over your mouth to the chin. The whole circuit takes fifteen to twenty seconds.

Eye-Socket Release

One of the face's favorite—but little-known—pockets of tension is the eye socket, just beneath the ridge of bone below the eyebrows. The key spot is where the ridge of bone meets the nose.

With your thumbs resting on the bone beneath each eyebrow, at the bridge of the nose—and being very careful not to press into the eyeball itself—massage in small circular strokes, pressing gently, for a minute or two.

Then lightly pinch the top of the bridge of the nose between your thumb and forefinger.

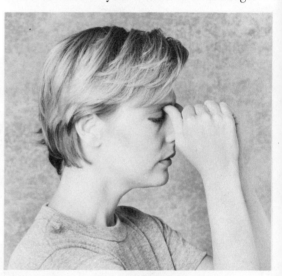

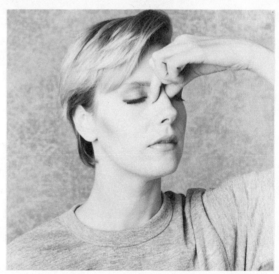

The Nose Job

With the forefingers of each hand, begin at the top of the nose and press firmly as you move down in small, circular strokes to the tip, then back again. Move out from the sides of the nose to massage the sinuses on either side.

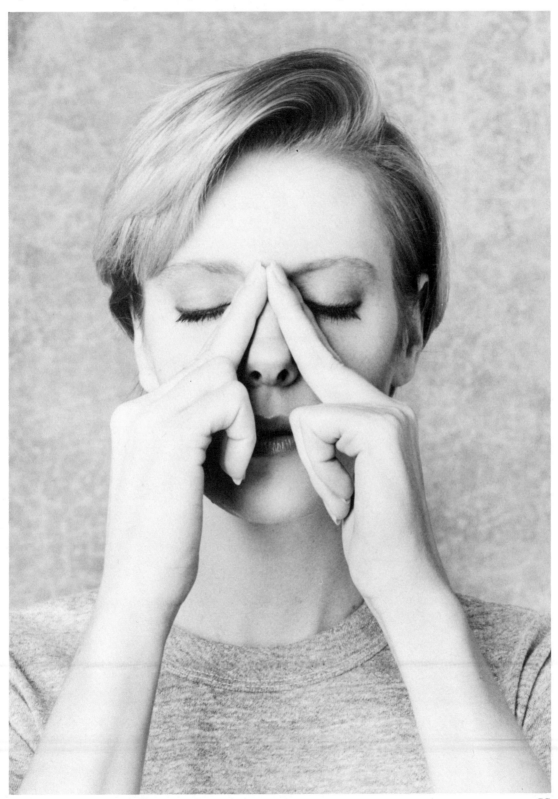

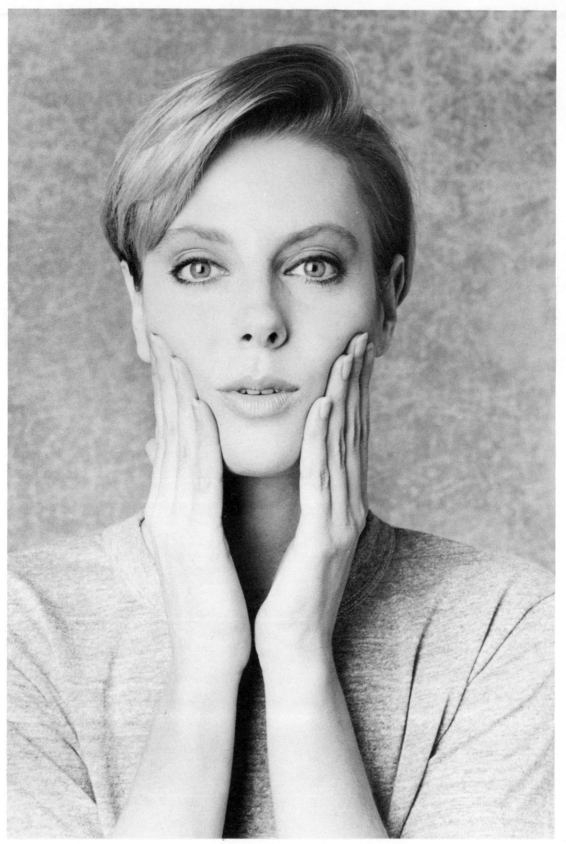

The Cheeks

Now use the same stroke with your fingertips to massage along the rim of bone beneath the eye sockets. Small, circular strokes work best. Focus on a small area, then move on to another.

Continue on to cover the whole surface of the cheeks, pressing firmly with your fingertips. Keep going down the face, including the upper lip and chin.

Ear Rubs

Don't forget your ears. They deserve a little attention. Start by rubbing your ears with your palms in a brisk up-and-down motion for ten to fifteen seconds. Then massage the lobes by pressing them firmly between thumb and forefinger. Go around the whole surface of the ear.

Finally, hold each earlobe between your thumb and forefinger, pinching firmly. Then gently tug at the lobe, stretching the ear. Work around the entire outer rim of the lobe.

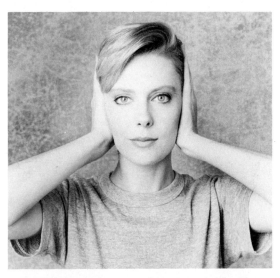

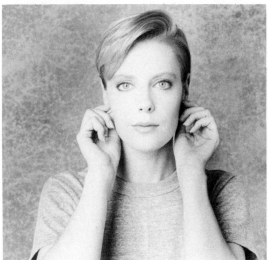

FACE MASSAGE FOR A FRIEND

There's something particularly soothing about a face massage. It's one of those special areas that, when completely relaxed, can induce an almost trancelike state of melting, total repose.

Let's say you want to give another person a massage. Have the person lie comfortably on his or her back and loosen any tight clothing. It's more comfortable for you to work from the top of the head.

To set the mood and help you both calm down a bit, simply put your palms lightly on the person's forehead, your palms almost meeting at the center, your fingers pointing out to the temples. Stay there quietly for a few moments to let the person get used to your touch and to focus your full awareness on what you're doing.

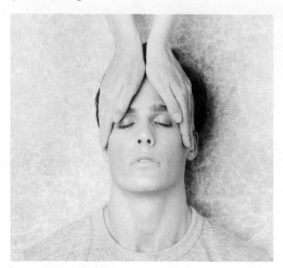

Scalp

Start here. Slide your hands onto the scalp and knead across the whole head of hair firmly with your fingertips. Work down to the side of the head and upper neck. Apply fingertips firmly to the scalp, not the hair. Move your fingers to a section of the scalp, press firmly in a circular movement, and then move to another area.

Be gentle. The receiver should not have to strain to oppose the force of your massage. If necessary, support the head with one hand while the other works the opposite side. And move with the grain of the hair so there is no tugging.

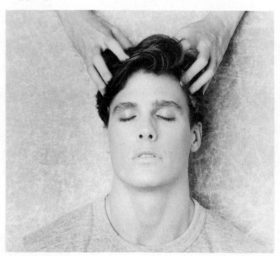

Forehead

Using your thumbs, start at the center of the forehead at the hairline. With about the pressure it takes to stick a stamp on an envelope, slide your thumbs out to the temples. End the stroke there with a circular rub. Then go back to the middle of the forehead, just below the last stroke, and slide out again toward the temples, using the same stroke. Work down to the eyebrows.

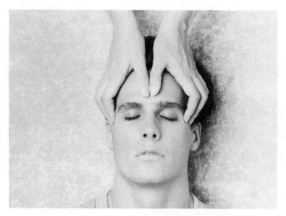

Eye Area

Using a light touch with your fingertips, trace the arc around the eye, from the top of the nose along the eyebrows, around the bottom of the socket, and back to the bridge of the nose. Do this a few times, and then place your thumbs on the bone beneath the brow so the thumb tips touch the bridge of the nose. Press here firmly for five or six seconds. (Stay clear of the eyeball.)

Finally, a delicate, featherlike stroke over the closed eyelids can be quite soothing. Be extra gentle—the skin here is quite sensitive, and the eye is just beneath. <u>Caution</u>: Don't do this if the person wears contact lenses.

Cheeks

Move your thumbs and fingertips down to the cheekbones and with a firm, circular stroke, massage the sides of the nose along the cheekbone to the ears. Spend extra time on the area where the cheekbones meet the nose, especially just above and to the sides of the nostrils. (But don't press the nostrils closed; it's hard to relax while suffocating.)

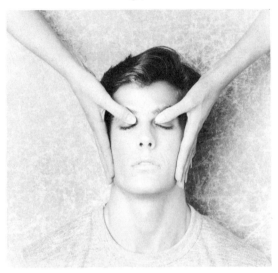

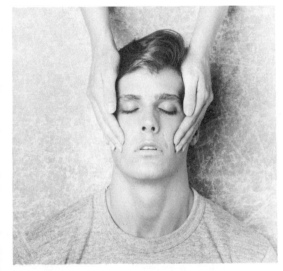

Jaw

With your fingertips, find the masseter, the broad muscle that extends from the jaw up to the cheekbone (see drawing). Use firm pressure to massage from just in front of the ears down along the jaw. Spend more time at the top of the jaw, where it hinges into the skull—it's the point just about in front of the earlobes.

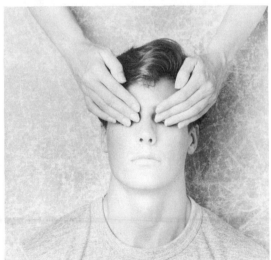

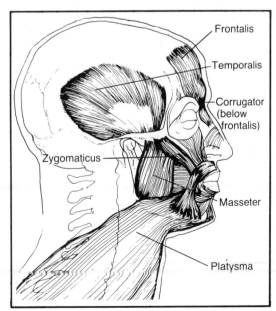

59

Chin

Use your forefingers to massage the chin in a stroke that follows the edge of the jaw from the tip of the chin almost up to the ears. With your fingertips, massage lightly around the mouth from the center of the chin to the upper lip. If the person being massaged has a beard, massage over it with firm strokes. Be sure to apply pressure directly to the skin to avoid pulling the hairs.

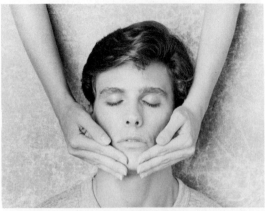

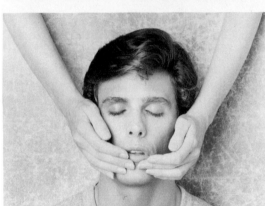

Ears

With your thumb and forefingers, work along the fleshy part of the earlobes and around the rims. The topography of the ear invites some free-form work. Just be gentle and slow.

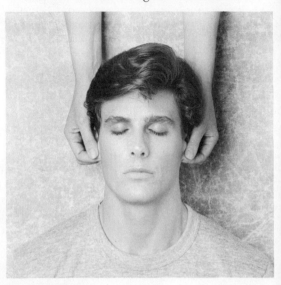

The End

Finish by using your whole open hand to stroke lightly over the entire face. Finally, place your open hands lightly over the receiver's closed eyes, your fingertips touching at the nose, palms out toward the ears. Rest there for several moments while you both relish the calm of a relaxed face.

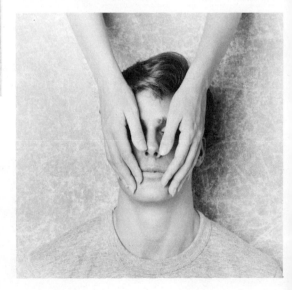

PRESSURE POINTS FOR TENSION RELIEF

The Oriental massage technique of acupressure uses fingertip presses on key points to relieve tension. The face has several such points, each of which offers some measure of quick relief for tension in that area.

Points to Press

1. Several key areas are located around the eye. Use your thumb in the notch just under the eyebrow at the point where the thumb rests against the side of the nose. Press here firmly for five to ten seconds. Then move out along the ridge of the bone, about a thumb's width, pressing each point. Close your eyes while you do this, but be careful not to press the eye itself.

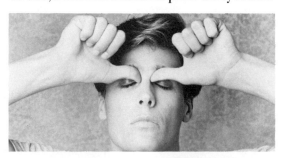

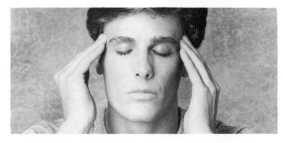

2. Follow the curve of the eye socket to the outer edge of the eye, and move toward the ear, about a finger's width, until you find a small pocket in the bone, near the temple. Press there with your fingertips.
3. Move fingers just below the nostrils, where you can feel your teeth begin in the skull. Press into the groove.

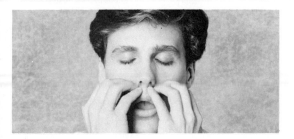

4. Find the small crevice just behind the earlobes. Use a softer, steady pressure here.

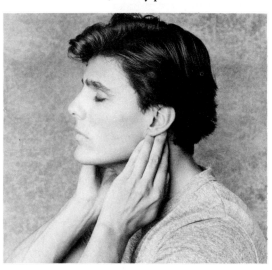

61

FACE TREATS

The facial, that standby of beauty treatments, can be a great relaxer. Like any application of wet heat, it draws the blood to the muscles of the face, helping flush the buildup of toxins.

Do-It-Yourself Facial

It's simple to give yourself a facial. All you need is a soft towel, some cotton pads with cleansing lotion, a facial mask, and an astringent. There are many masks available—ginseng texturizing masks and clay, vegetable, and herbal masks, among others. All these products can be found at cosmetic counters or natural-food stores.

Step 1. Wash your face thoroughly in mild soap and water, then pat it dry with a soft towel.

Step 2. Clean your face with cotton pads and cleansing lotion.

Step 3. Apply the mask, following its specific directions.

Step 4. After you've removed the mask, bask a while with a hot, steaming towel covering your face. Arrange the towel around your nose so you can breathe. In addition, an extra small, moist cloth—or folded paper towel—placed over each eye is especially soothing.

Step 5. Finally, if you like, apply a gentle astringent to close the pores.

Face Bonus

To bring the blood to your face, a rubber complexion brush does wonders in a jiffy. Or try a slant board. The tilt will bring blood to your face and reverse the pull of gravity on facial muscles.

There you are. Massaged, pampered, serene, and relaxed. Stretch, *purrrr*—and off you go to face the world.

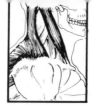

Chapter 7

Necksavers

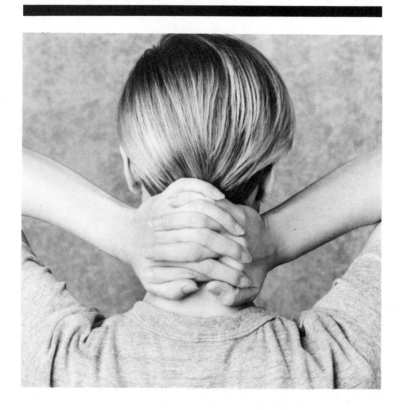

The trunk of the body, mainly the neck and back, is a primary target for user-nasty office equipment, procrustean furniture, and unanatomical car seats. In addition, mental tension readily expresses itself in hardworking neck muscles. Most of us who get a stiff neck simply put up with the pain and loss of movement, hoping it will go away by itself. It usually does—in a week or two. But if you know how to unknot that pain in the neck, recovery can be a matter of days, even hours.

If pain is bad or persistent, of course, see your doctor. But for cricks, knots, and other everyday agonies, here's an assortment of easy necksoothers. Some are quick fixes, others offer long-term relief and prevention. Make your own mix.

KNOW YOUR NECK

The neck actually consists of the seven loosely joined cervical vertebrae at the top of the spine. The spine is near the center of the neck, not at the back as many of us imagine. This neck section of the spinal column is wrapped in dozens of muscles that contract and relax every time you move your head or alter the alignment of spine and skull. These muscles have a tricky engineering job, a little like balancing a wobbling melon on a broomstick.

The most vulnerable neck muscle is the *trapezius*. It runs from the base of the skull down the back of the neck, where it fans out to the shoulder blades and spine. Slumping or carrying your head too far forward strains this muscle. "Slump" may sound relaxed; actually, it's just the opposite—body talk for the intense, hardworking lives we live. Working all day at a desk, typing, and tracking the video screen of a word processor or computer foster poor head posture and overtime for the trapezius.

Wearing high heels also strains this muscle. The heels pitch a woman's legs forward, thrusting her buttocks back. To compensate for this architectural realignment, chest, neck, and head tilt forward. But this means the trapezius must strain to hold the head in place.

The other major pain-in-the neck muscle is the *sternomastoid*. To find it, turn your head toward your shoulder and run your hand along the protruding muscle that extends from the base of the skull just below the ear down the front of the neck to your collarbone. The sternomastoid supports the neck to the side and front, whereas the trapezius controls front and back. If you brace your shoulder against a heavy shoulder bag, strain while lugging a suitcase, or scrunch up to the telephone receiver, you tense both the trapezius and sternomastoid.

Mental stress can create or compound neck pain. If you are depressed or angry, your muscles may tense without your noticing. The longer the tension holds, the more likely the muscle will harden into a painful knot.

The key to breaking the spasm-pain cycle is to relax the muscle and increase circulation. A hot bath or heating pad will help. And so will gentle massage and other simple exercises. Find the combination that suits your neck. Relax and enjoy yourself.

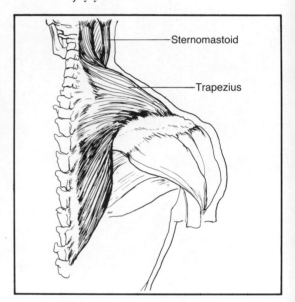

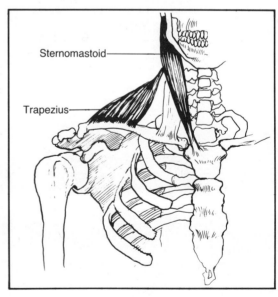

SAVE YOUR NECK

 Heat. Remember, heat soothes and heals. To get heat to your neck, try any of the following:

■ Stand in a comfortably warm shower with a towel over the section that hurts. Let the warm water soak the towel, which, in turn, will maintain even, comfortable heat. Or relax in a deep, warm bath.

■ Set a heating pad on low and place it directly over the problem area. Try it for twenty minutes, and repeat every hour or so as needed.

■ Use a hot-water bottle wrapped in a moist washcloth. Moist heat is better than dry heat.

Massage. Massage can bring immediate relief to neck aches. If a caring friend will help, wonderful. But you can do a lot for yourself. Work down or up from the end toward the belly of the muscle. If you press too hard in the middle of a muscle in spasm, the spasm may get worse. And any time you feel a sharp pain as you massage, ease up.

Pressure-Point Massage

This Japanese adaptation of acupuncture uses finger pressure on key points of energy flow. With your middle fingers, find the bumps at the base of your skull just below your ears. Press your fingers on the sternomastoid as it connects to these bumps. Press firmly and steadily for five to ten seconds, then release. Repeat.

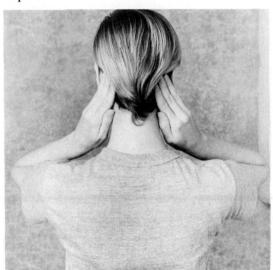

Pinpoint Massage

With one hand, reach back and find the trapezius muscle. Remember, it runs along your spine from the top of your neck to your shoulder blade. Beginning at the shoulder blade and following it along the spine to your skull, work it with your fingertips, using a small, circular motion. Switch hands and repeat on the other side.

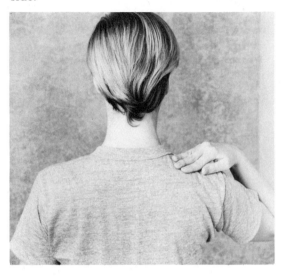

Palms On

Clasp your hands behind your neck and knead the trapezius with the heels of your palms.

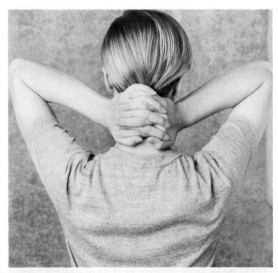

Easy Neck Stretches

 Slow, gentle movements help tight muscles regain flexibility. Do these neck stretches in a comfortable sitting position, with your shoulders relaxed. The number of repetitions is up to you. Five times is fine; more if you wish.

Side Stretch

With your shoulders relaxed, tilt your head so your left ear reaches toward your shoulder. Feel the stretch. Then repeat on the right.

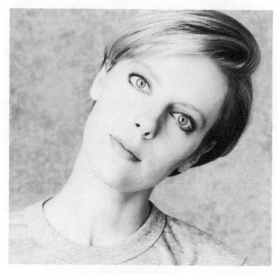

Over-the-Shoulder Stretch

Turn your head slowly and look over your left shoulder. Feel the stretch; repeat on the right.

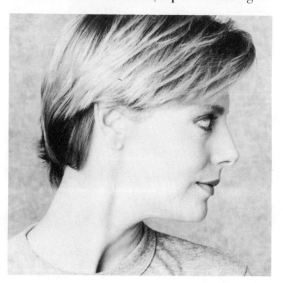

Caution: Whether changing a light bulb or doing a neck roll, don't tilt your head back too far. The head is very heavy. Resting on the base of the neck, it's well supported. But the more it rocks from atop the first vertebra, the more strain. When you look up at the ceiling tilting your head back, you compress the neck vertebrae, overstretch the muscle at the front of the neck, and tense those in the neck and shoulders. Here are two solutions:

1. When doing neck rotations, roll up a towel and drape it over the base of your neck. The towel roll will support and cushion your head as it rolls back.

2. Instead or rotating your head in a circle, try an oval, with the far points at the sides.

Jaw Stretch

Read <u>Caution</u> above. Then let your head drop forward, your chin reaching toward your chest. Hold for a few moments without tensing. Now lift your head and gently let it fall back—but not all the way. Slowly let your jaw open and relax. Repeat.

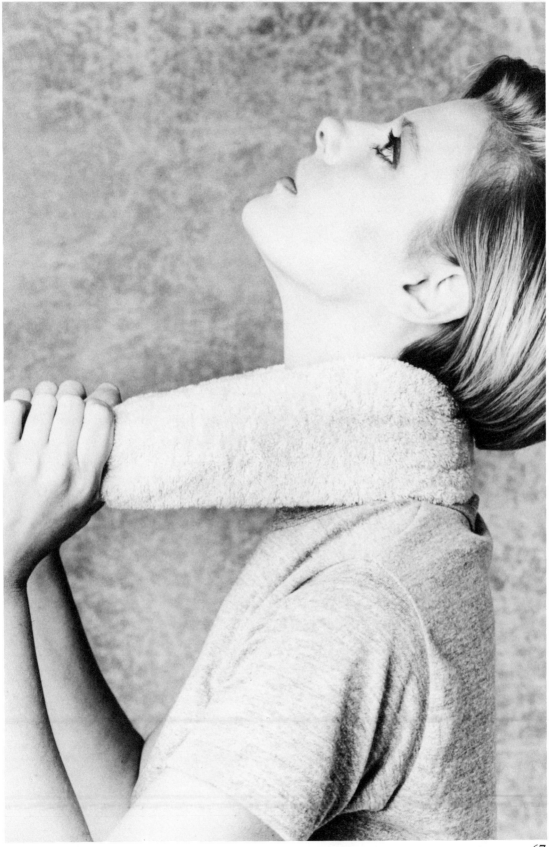

Revolving Stretch

Read Caution, p.66. Start with your head dropped on your chest. Slowly rotate it around to the right, the back (don't let it drop), the left, and back to the front. Then switch directions. If you feel points of tension, pause a moment and let those muscles relax. If you feel an excess of cracking, stop. Try the bobbing stretch instead.

Bobbing Stretch

Instead of revolving your neck, go from an upright position to each of the four positions—right, back, left, front—but return to the upright position in between.

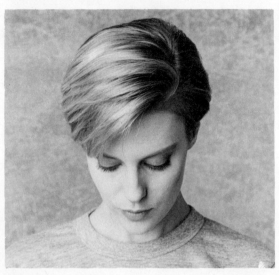

Clock Stretch I

Imagine you're looking at a clockface. Move your neck to the left, toward 9 o'clock, then to the right, toward 3. Then up toward 12 and down to 6. Repeat these three times in each direction.

Clock Stretch II

Now face up toward the left at a forty-five-degree angle, then up to the right at the same angle. Next, down forty-five degrees to the left, then right. Repeat.

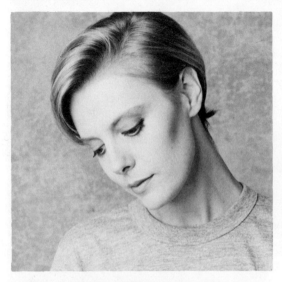

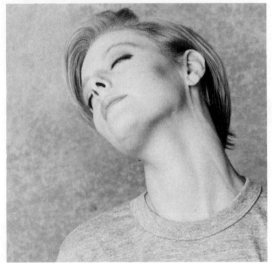

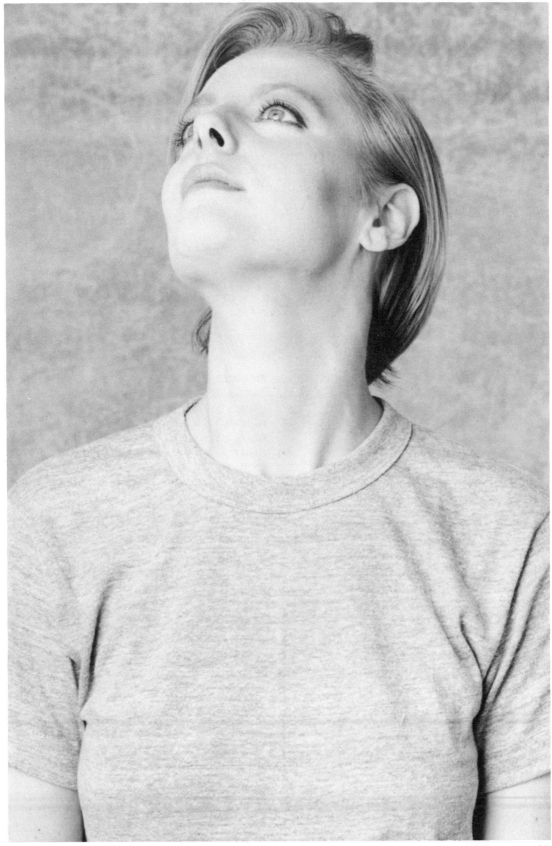

More Stretches

Arm Stretch

This move relaxes your poor, strained sterno-mastoid. Put your right arm behind your back and grasp your wrist with your left hand. Gently pull your right arm down and across your back while you lean your head toward the left. Feel a comfortable stretch down your neck and side while you hold the position ten to fifteen seconds. Repeat two or three times on both sides.

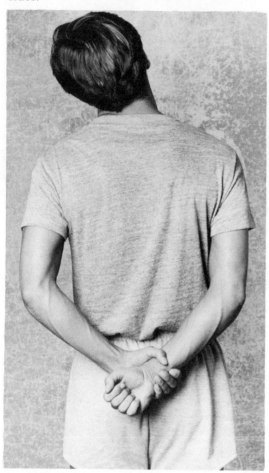

Now spread a folded blanket or mat on the floor and make yourself comfortable. Here are two stretches that relieve the trapezius, easing pain ascending from the upper back to the neck.

Bending Stretch I

Lie on your back with your knees raised, feet on the floor. Lock your fingers behind your ears. Exhale while you pull up with your arms and slowly bend your head forward. Stay there for about five seconds. Feel the slight stretch at the back of your neck. Slowly lower your head to the floor, inhaling. Repeat three times.

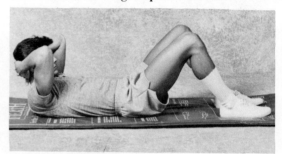

Bending Stretch II

Assume the same position on the floor and clasp your hands behind your ears. But this time exhale and pull up so your chin points toward your left knee. Hold it five seconds, then lower your head to the floor. Breathe naturally and r-e-l-a-x. Then repeat the exercise toward your right knee. Try this three times to each side.

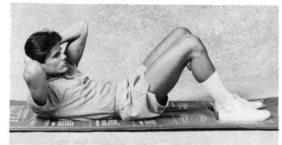

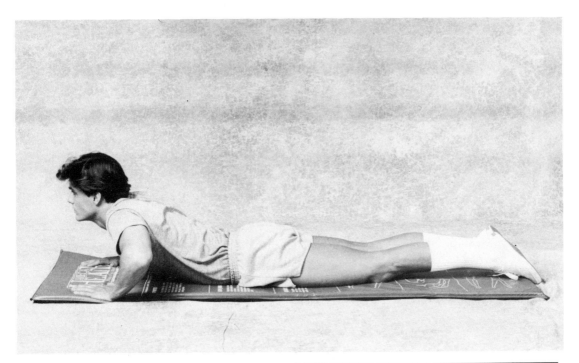

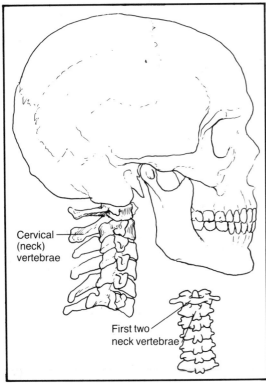

Cervical (neck) vertebrae

First two neck vertebrae

MOVES FOR AWARENESS

■ Lie on your stomach with your forehead to the floor. Place your hands on the floor beside your shoulders, pointing toward your head. Elbows should be bent, palms turned down.

Very gently raise your head and shoulders from the floor, leaning backward. Your back should arch gently, your stomach and lower chest remaining on the floor. Then lower your body back to the floor and rest. Repeat three or four times.

■ Turn over on your back and roll your head gently from side to side. Be especially attuned to the movements of your neck muscles as your head rocks. Go slowly and be aware of points of tension: Is one side worse than the other?

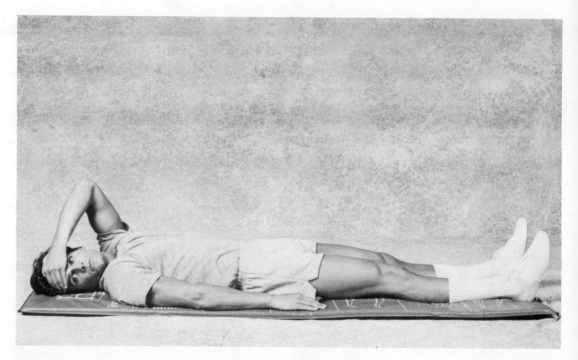

■ Still lying on your back, rest your left hand on your forehead so you feel its full weight. Use your hand to guide your head from side to side. Let your head be lazy and heavy. Your hand does all the work: Push your head to the right with your palm; pull it to the left with your fingers. Repeat slowly several times. Then do the same using your right hand.

■ Now roll over to the position you began with. Starting with your forehead on the floor, move your head until your chin rests on the floor. Hold this position while you run your eyes along the floor until you see the wall in front of you. Fix your gaze at that point for a few moments and bring your forehead back to the floor. Repeat this motion several times, slowly.

Don't hold your breath; breathe naturally and be aware of the sensations in your neck and shoulder blades. Try to picture your spine as you move.

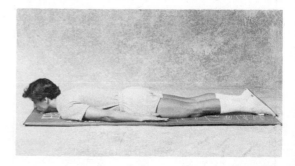

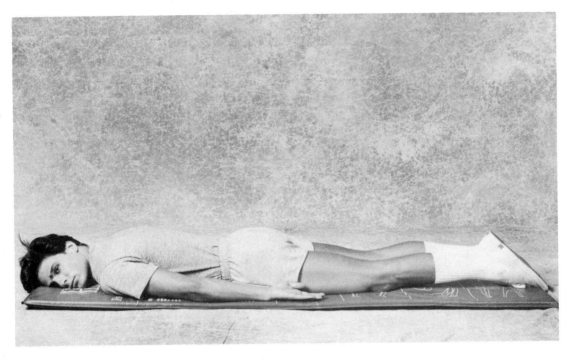

■ Still on your stomach, turn your face to the left so your left ear rests on the floor. Slowly move your head till your forehead rests on the floor. Gently repeat this movement several times. Now turn your face to the right and repeat exercise.

YOGA BREATHING MOVES

Coordinating your breathing and neck movements enhances relaxation. Always keep in mind the basic yoga principle: Exhale as you fold your body, inhale as you open it.

Try to be aware of your breathing pattern as you do the following neck movements:

■ Sit comfortably in a chair. If you can, roll your tongue in a furrow so you can breathe through it like a straw (or purse your lips). Tip your head back as you inhale through your tongue. (Remember, don't tilt too far backward.) Then exhale as you bring your head down toward your chest. Repeat. Be gentle. Don't jam your head against your back and chest, but stop at a comfortable point.

■ Get on your hands and knees. Lift your head up and arch your back, inhaling as you make the movement. Round your back and drop your head as you exhale. Repeat.

PREVENTION

Most neck knots are preventable. One way to ward off pain is to notice—and break—the physical habits that tighten neck muscles.

■ If you carry a heavy shoulder bag or briefcase, switch sides often and support the strap with your hand at the shoulder. Better still, switch to a backpack to even out the load. Besides, do you really have to cart all that stuff home every night?

■ If you jam a phone between your neck and shoulders, buy a shoulder rest or hold it with your hand.

■ On supertense days, pause to notice whether your neck muscles feel tight. If so, take a few minutes to do some exercises. Heeding an early-warning system is the best way to head off tension buildup.

■ Don't slump. Remind yourself to keep your back, neck, and head aligned, especially if you work long hours at a typewriter or computer terminal. But be gentle with your body. Sitting ramrod straight doesn't help. If your word processor is also processing you, you may need special help. Chapter 14, "Pain in the Office," p.59, offers more detailed survival tips.

■ Watch out for deadly desks. Take a few minutes now and then to release the tension buildup. Be aware of your usual neck positions and change them:

1. Take a break. Walk around, stretching your arms to get more blood to your shoulders and neck.

2. Tailor your chair to your back. Placing a small pillow at your lower back may help.

3. Get your neck moving. Sitting at your desk, let your arms hang loose to the sides. If your chair has arms, sit toward the front. Now lift your shoulders toward your ears, inhaling deeply. Hold them up for a count of five.

Drop your shoulders, exhaling deeply. Let your arms hang to the sides, feeling them as heavy and warm.

Slowly roll your shoulders, five times to the front, five times to the back.

4. Place your left hand on your right shoulder so the fingers touch the trapezius at the top and back. Press into the muscle and massage. Switch arms and massage the other side.

5. Now put both hands on opposite shoulders so they cross at your chest. Relax your shoulder muscles—let them drop—and slowly roll your head in an oval, taking care not to let it drop back. Reverse direction.

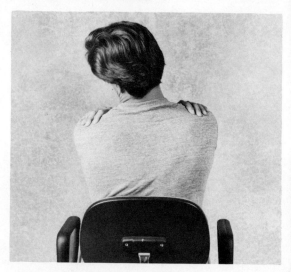

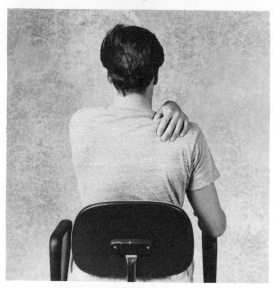

AWARENESS TIPS

■ Many of us tend to lead movements from the chin. This pulls the head back and down, tensing the muscles at the back of the neck. To prevent this, think of your chin as part of your head—not a ship's prow.

■ While talking, there's a tendency to tighten the head back and lower the chin toward the chest, tensing the neck muscles. If you feel tension around your neck when talking, try to let your head rise as though it were being pulled upward by a string.

■ When sitting at a desk or reading, try not to slouch forward; it strains the back of the neck. When you find yourself doing this, sit up straight—but not stiff—and reposition your head so it rests squarely atop your neck.

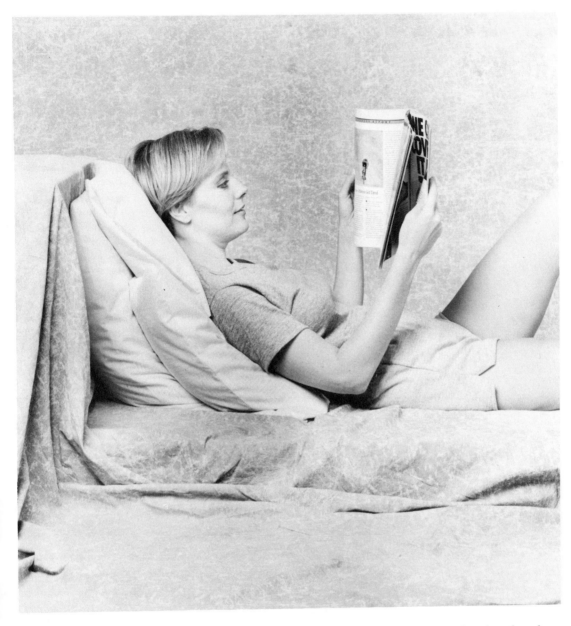

PILLOW TALK

Curling up in bed at night may relax the inner you, but it can be hard work for your neck muscles. Here are some basic guidelines for preventing neck strain while you sleep.

■ Use a firm mattress.

■ When you lie on your back, support your head with a single small pillow to relieve neck strain. Heaping pillows high puts too much stress on your neck. One pillow minimizes pressure on the neck.

■ When you lie on your side, place a fat pillow (or two pillows) under your head and neck so that your ribs—instead of shoulders and neck—support more of your upper body weight.

■ Reading or watching TV in bed can be a real pain in the neck. It doesn't have to be.

The Wrong Way. Don't lie with support under only one part of your head or neck. This supports one muscle group but it strains the others.

The Right Way. Support the entire neck and upper shoulders. Use enough pillows to provide support from the shoulders all the way up the neck to the top of the head.

MIND OVER MUSCLE

In their rhythms of tensing and relaxing, your muscles mirror your mind. If you are relaxed, your muscles will be, too. The following mental exercises will ease neck pain and make your neck muscles more flexible.

■ Sit forward on a firm chair, balancing your weight on the bony protuberances in your buttocks—your "sit bones." Now imagine a string attached to your head gently pulling you upward. Sense the upward pull while you sit still for five or ten seconds. This will help stretch your spine.

■ Imagine you're a mandarin doll with a rocking head, and let your head rock up and down in small movements until it comes to rest in a balanced, easy position, with minimal strain on your neck.

■ The first vertebra and the bottom of the skull act like a ring around a rod. Visualize these bones between your earlobes. Now, in small movements, move your head gently from side to side. Let the ring bone turn around the rod.

■ Imagine your neck as a wrinkled collar. Visualize the wrinkles smoothing out, starting from the lower collar at the base of the neck to the upper collar at the base of the skull.

■ With your fingers, find the indentation behind your ears. Imagine these spaces on each side of the head moving apart, enlarging the head space between them.

These simple exercises train the neck to use the smaller muscles that support the spine, rather than the larger muscles at the surface, which control grosser movement. Fine-tuning these inner muscles relaxes the larger muscles—which are more prone to ache.

Remember, it's your neck—supporting your head—that takes a beating as you "head" into your daily schedule. So give your neck a real break. To head off knots and muscle spasm, pause regularly to do a few neck-savers—quick stretches, spot massages—and be alert to the physical habits that abuse this hardworking set of muscles.

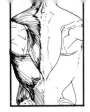

Chapter 8

Backsavers:
Six Weeks
to a
Healthy Back

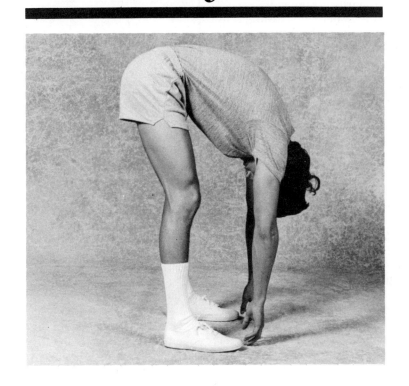

The backsaver exercises—bend, stretch, flex—in this chapter, the first of two devoted to back care, may not *sound* relaxing. But, in fact, building strength and flexibility is the key to relaxation in this region of your body. A strong back also guarantees decent working conditions for outlying muscles required to pinch-hit for out-of-whack back-support muscles. (Not all the back muscles are in the back.) Thus, building a strong back is a wise preventive measure, since weak muscles must contract and tense more than strong ones. This not only causes pain and spasm in the muscles that support the back, but creates tension in the rest of the body.

If you already have back problems, these exercises may be just what you need, but check with your doctor before you embark on this six-week course. This chapter will show you how to stress-proof your back by strengthening it; the next chapter, "Backsoothers," tenders loving care for hardworking muscles subjected to the inevitable demands of everyday stress. But first, let's inspect the anatomy of the human back—an engineering marvel and a potential disaster.

KNOW YOUR BACK

The bones, muscles, and other components of the human back evolved as a clever solution to a complex anatomical problem. A soft-fleshed, defenseless creature like a human being requires a flexible back that allows it to twist and wriggle out of danger and turn its head quickly. But the back must be rigid enough to help protect and support vulnerable internal organs and house the spinal cord, the main stem of the nervous system that links brain and body. Finally, it supports the delicate brain itself, which must be cushioned from the jolts and jars of living.

Nature's answer to these demands is the backbone, flexible in some places and rigid in others. Your spine is composed of a stack of smaller bones, the vertebrae, with disk-shaped cushions in between. Each vertebra (from the Latin *vertere*, to turn) has a hole through which the spinal cord passes, like a string through a necklace of pearls. How well your back serves you depends on how well it is maintained. As we get older, it becomes increasingly important to keep the back muscles fit; doctors estimate that 95 percent of all back problems are muscular. And the muscles that lead to most backaches aren't in the back at all.

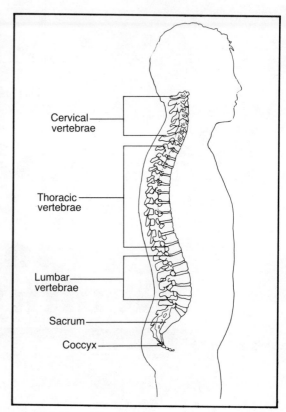

Cervical vertebrae

Thoracic vertebrae

Lumbar vertebrae

Sacrum

Coccyx

At the top of the S-curved spine there are seven loosely joined cervical (neck) vertebrae; the twelve thoracic vertebrae below them form the rigid rear of the rib cage. Then come the five vertebrae of the flexible lumbar region. At the crucial junction with the ileum, at the rear of the pelvis, the five sacral vertebrae are fused into a single bone. These lower-back areas are notorious for painful "lumbago" and "sacroiliac" problems. At the base of the spine the remaining three or four vertebrae are fused to form the coccyx, or tailbone.

The vertebrae account for only 75 percent of the length of the spine. The rest is made up of disks—fibrous pads between the vertebrae that make room for nerves branching from the spinal cord and extending to outlying parts of the body. Each disk is shaped to tilt the adjacent vertebrae backward or forward and give the backbone its overall S curve. Like the coils of a spring, the curves of the spine provide a little "give," protecting the brain from jolts or concussion.

To enhance the shock-absorber effect, each disk has a soft, pulpy inner core. In youngsters this stuffing is nearly all water; by age seventy the pulpy material loses 30 percent of its water content. As the disks thin with age, the spine can lose an inch or more of its length.

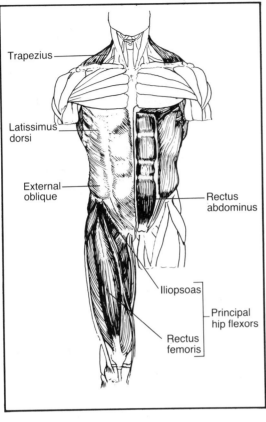

Trapezius

Latissimus dorsi

External oblique

Rectus abdominus

Iliopsoas

Principal hip flexors

Rectus femoris

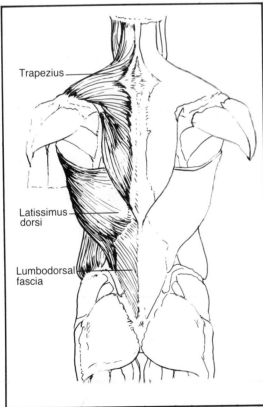

Trapezius

Latissimus dorsi

Lumbodorsal fascia

Three main sets of muscles work with the backbone. Those along each side of the spine—trapezius, lumbodorsal fascia, latissimus dorsi—keep the backbone erect and enable you to bend backward. The hip flexors raise the thigh as you step forward. And the abdominal muscles, running from groin to chest, bend you forward in the classic sit-up motion. When weak abdominal muscles and hip flexors abdicate their responsibilities—a risk that increases after the age of forty—the job of holding you suitably erect falls entirely to the back muscles, which protest with tension and pain.

The back is also prey to muscle spasms triggered by tension and emotional stress—worse if muscles are weak. Because of the enormous physical demands made on the back, it's important to strengthen these muscles through exercise. Remember, when a muscle tenses, it loses its stretch and eventually shortens. A permanently contracted muscle is always on the verge of spasm and can no longer relax. If your back muscles have reached this state, you may be prone to backaches.

But training can build strength and restore elasticity to your back muscles. And as you rebuild your abdominals and hip flexors, you take much of the strain off the actual back muscles. A strong muscle, it's important to remember, can be a relaxed muscle, too. Building muscles that can tense when called upon and then relax is the goal of the six-week backsaver regimen that follows.

THE STATE-OF-YOUR-BACK TEST

Before you start your exercise program, try this simple diagnostic test to detect muscle groups that may need special attention. Once you start the backsaver exercises, the test can be used every week to chart your progress. Chronic back woes may stem from any of several deficiencies, including underpowered hip flexors, flabby stomach muscles, and too-taut back muscles. Knowing your main weak spots will help you focus on those areas as you go through the backsaver regimen.

To start, get comfortable. Remove your shoes, loosen any tight clothing, and take a few moments to let your mind calm down. Do each test slowly and deliberately; don't strain. These are diagnostic tests for you alone.

If you have a chronic back condition, check with your physician first before trying the test—or the backsaver routine. And remember, as always, if it hurts, stop at once.

Hip-Flexor Test

Lie on your back and clasp your hands behind your neck with your legs together, out straight. Keeping your knees straight, lift your feet till your heels are about ten inches from the floor. Try to hold for a slow count of ten. If you have to drop your legs before the count is up, your hips need strengthening.

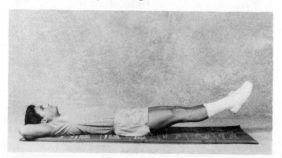

Hip and Stomach Test

Lying flat on the floor, your hands still clasped behind your neck, protect your back by anchoring your feet under a heavy piece of furniture or ask a friend to hold your ankles. Now do a single sit-up. If you can do one sit-up, you've passed. If not, it means your hip flexors and stomach muscles cannot support your trunk. You should focus on both these areas.

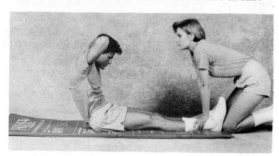

Stomach Test

Get in the same position, but with your knees flexed, your heels close to your bottom. Try another sit-up. Can't do it? Then work on those stomach muscles.

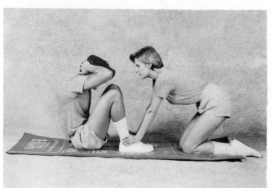

Back-Muscle Test

You'll need a helper for this one. Turn face down, with a pillow under your stomach. Ask your helper to put one hand on your lower back, the other on your ankles, and to hold you steady while you lift your trunk. Hold the position for a slow count of ten. If you can't, your back muscles need strengthening.

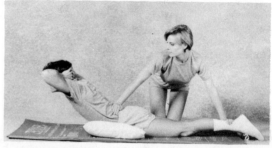

Lower-Back Test

In the same position, with your arms folded under your head, have your helper hold your back steady. Now lift your legs, keeping your knees straight, and hold the position for ten seconds. If you had to drop your legs, your lower-back muscles need work.

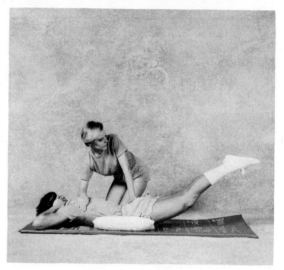

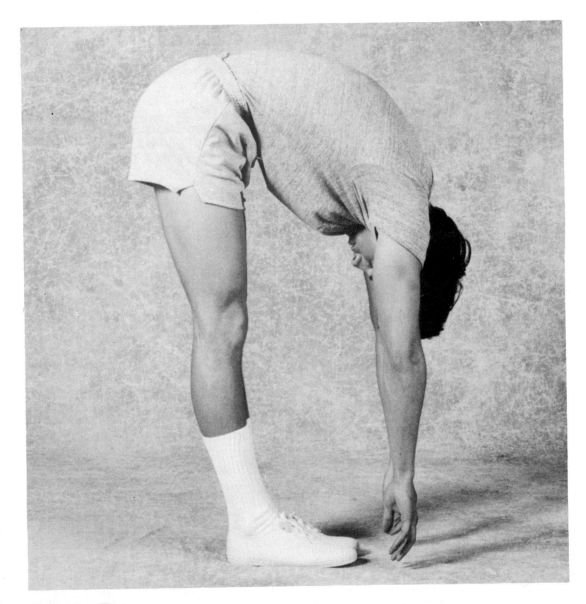

Hamstring Test

Finally, stand up straight, feet together. Slowly, gently lean over and touch the floor with your fingertips, keeping your legs straight. If you can do it, congratulations! If not, tension is shortening your back muscles and hamstrings, the tendons and muscles at the back of your thighs.

SIX-WEEK BACKSAVER REGIMEN

Now that you know where the problems are, you're ready to go to work. Remember that though you're about to embark on a muscle-strengthening routine, the pursuit of a truly relaxed body requires a set of back muscles that can bear their share of the burden without going into spasm and without straining other muscles.

Here are eighteen gentle moves that may be used to repair ordinary aching backs and, even better, to head off problems before they develop. The course and the preceding test are adapted from the classic Kraus exercises by Alexander Melleby, a protege of back-exercise pioneer Dr. Hans Kraus. You'll find this six-week backsaver routine easy and nonstrenuous, but it's possible to overdo the exercises. If you have a back problem, get your doctor's OK first. Don't strain or rush. Do the exercises slowly and smoothly, without jerking or bouncing. Remember, a relaxed, flexible back is your goal; you're not planning to lift a piano. If any exercise hurts, skip it for two weeks.

Don't try all the exercises the first time. Start with the first six, the *relaxercises*. Work from numbers 1 to 6, doing each only three times. Then work back down from numbers 6 to 1. This assures that you really relax at the beginning and the end of each session. After four days, add numbers 7 and 8, and then back down. The first week's workout should take fifteen minutes.

At the start of the second week, add number 9; four days later, add number 10. From then on, add a new exercise at the beginning of each week, another four days later. It should take the full six weeks to work up to number 18. If your self-test has highlighted a special weak spot, you can alter the sequence a bit to concentrate on that area.

1. Basic Flat-on-Back Position. Lie on your back, arms at sides, knees bent, with feet flat on the floor or mat. Breathe deeply and close your eyes. Concentrate on relaxing throughout the first six exercises.

Limber Legs. Now slide one leg forward till it is flat on the floor. Slowly drag it back to the basic position. Do the other leg.

Limber Arms. Bend one arm at the elbow and let it drop to the floor. Now the other arm.

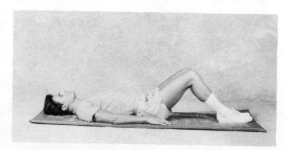

2. Prone Shrug. From the basic position, slide your shoulders up to your ears without lifting them from the floor. Return . . . repeat.

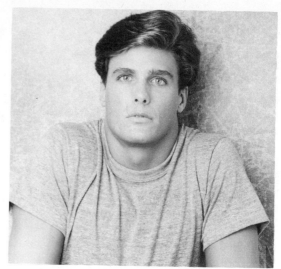

3. Basic Head Roll. From the basic position, let your head roll to one side. Now slowly roll it to the opposite side. Repeat.

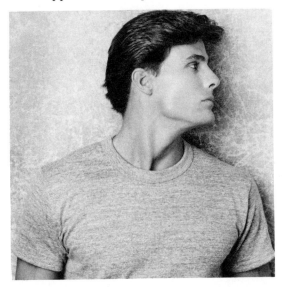

4. Knee Flex. From the basic position, slowly bring one knee up toward the shoulder, then return your foot to the mat and slide the leg out straight. Return to the basic position and repeat with the other leg.

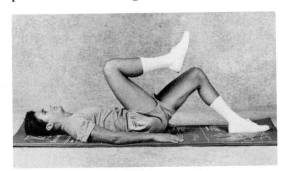

5. Fetal Leg Slide. Lie on your right side and curl your body into the fetal position with your head resting comfortably on your arm. Place the other arm in front or on your hip. Slide the top leg (consider it dead weight) up toward your shoulder, letting it fall off the lower leg. Now slide the leg out in a straight line and return to the fetal position. Repeat. Then roll over for the other leg.

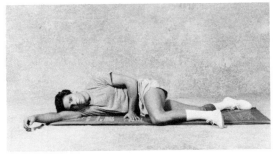

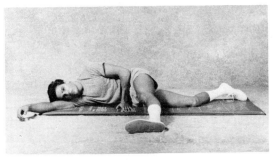

6. Squeeze Play. Lie on your stomach with your forehead resting on folded hands. Point your toes inward, exhale, and tighten your seat muscles. Hold two seconds and release, then repeat. You can actually do the muscle squeeze secretly at any time, in any position.

7. Double Knee Flex. From the basic position, pull both knees up to your chest, then gradually lower them as you return to the basic position. To give your abdominal muscles a good workout, hold your hips flat on the floor. Repeat, but do not do this or any other exercise more than three times in sequence.

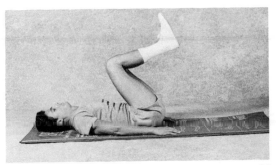

8. Cat Back. Kneel on all fours. Now arch your back like a cat; drop your head slowly and tuck your pelvis in. Reverse the exercise slowly, letting your stomach slump into a U. Raise your head and push your buttocks out at the same time. Repeat.

9. Half Sit-up. From the basic flat-on-back position, curl up to a half sit-up, bringing your fingertips to the top of your knees. Lower slowly and relax, then repeat. Notice that you are moving from flexibility exercises into muscle strengthening.

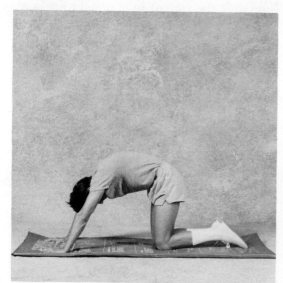

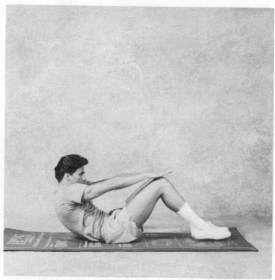

10. Praying Mantis. Turn over on your hands and knees. Place your hands and then your forearms on the ground. Keeping your thighs at a right angle to the mat, slide or walk your forearms forward while keeping your back and head straight. As soon as you feel a pull in the upper chest (pectoral muscles), slide or walk your forearms back to the start. Repeat.

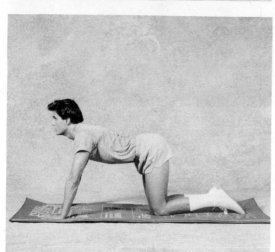

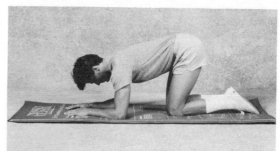

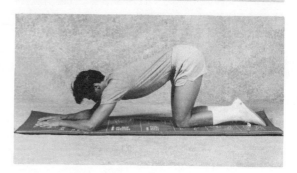

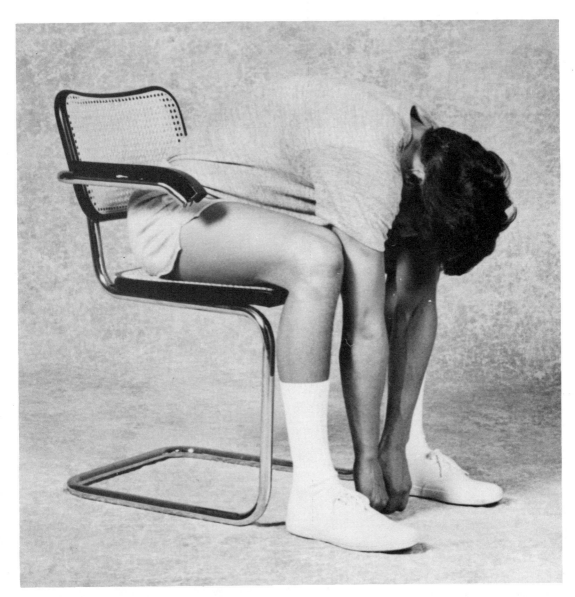

11. Chair Bend. Sit forward on a sturdy chair so that part of your weight rests on your feet and legs. Spread your legs, leaving space for your head and arms. Now slowly bend toward the floor by letting your chin drop to your chest and your shoulders sag. Let your shoulders come between your knees, arms dangling. Hang loose five seconds. Return, relax, repeat.

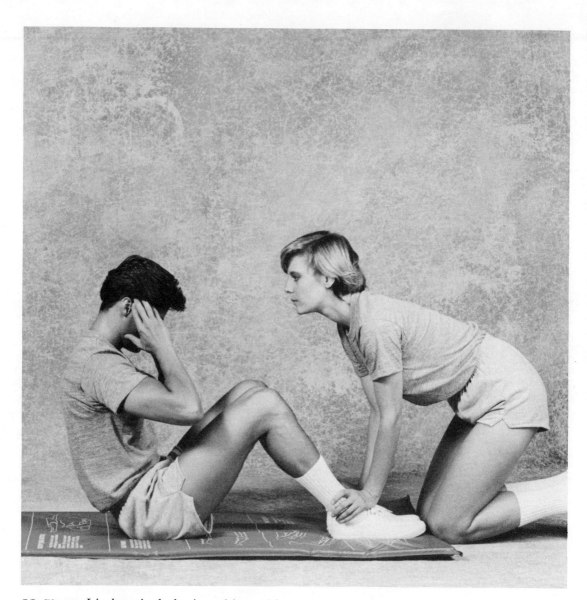

12. Sit-up. Lie down in the basic position, with your feet braced under a heavy object and your hands up beside your head. Do not put your hands behind your neck and snap yourself up. Roll up gently to a sitting position, as if lifting one vertebra at a time. Then slowly uncurl back down and relax. Repeat.

Hand Leverage. If your abdominal muscles are still too weak for a full sit-up, try it with your hands at your sides. As it gets easier, move your hands to your stomach, then your chest and head.

13. Chair Side-Straddle. Sit forward on a chair with your legs only slightly spread. To start, bring your arms straight over your head, then bring them forward and lower them to the right side toward the floor. When you have come down as far as you can with your chin near your knee and your arms at the side of your leg, hold for five seconds. Don't bounce. Now come up slowly . . . slide your arms across your lap and down again, this time to the left side.

14. Leg Stretcher. From the basic position, bring one knee up toward your chest, then extend the leg toward the ceiling. Point your toes straight up. With the leg fully extended, lower it slowly to the floor; then bend it back to the basic position. Now the other leg. Repeat, this time with the foot flexed, as if walking on the ceiling.

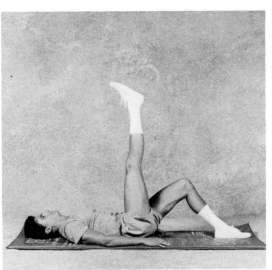

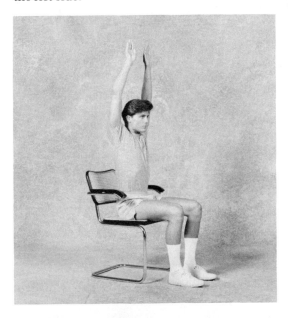

15. Hamstring Stretch. The hamstrings are tendons and muscles at the back of your thighs. From the basic position, slide your right leg forward, pointing your toes. With the knee locked, slowly raise the leg as high as you can. Lower it to the floor and drag your foot back to the start. Do the other leg. Now repeat with the foot flexed.

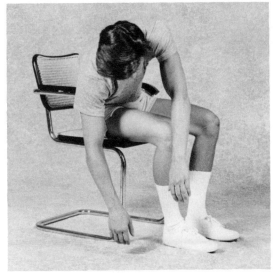

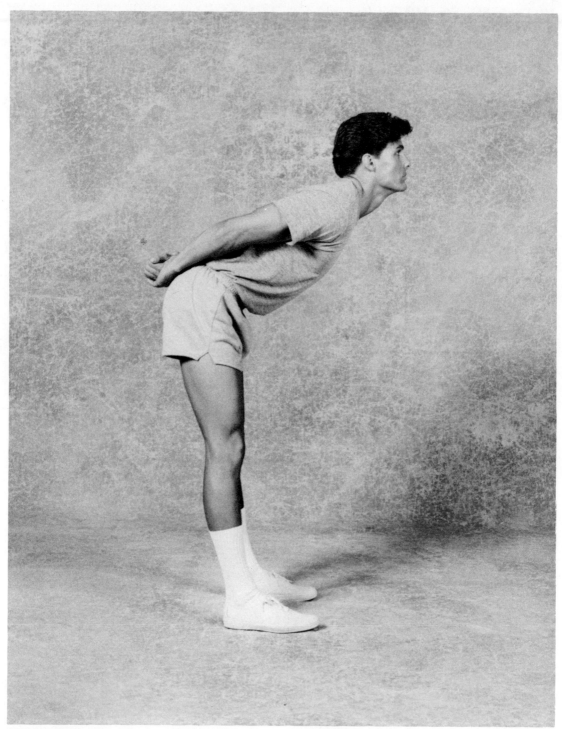

16. Rooster Stretch. Stand up and spread your legs apart. Put your arms behind your back and clasp your hands. Lock your elbows. Now slowly bend forward from the waist, keeping your head up. Bend forward until you can feel stretching in the back of your knees. Hold two seconds—straighten up, relax, and repeat.

17. Calf Stretch. Face a wall at arm's length with your feet together and hips straight. Place your hands flat on the wall. Without lifting your heels or bending from the waist, lean toward the wall. Bend your arms at the elbow until your arms come in contact with it. Then use your arms to push your body back. Repeat.

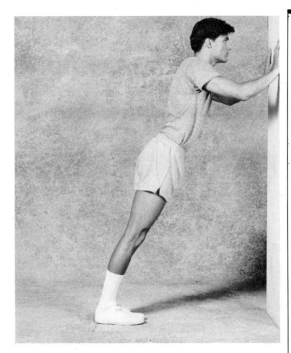

18. Double Over. Stand up straight, legs apart. Keeping your knees as straight as possible (but don't lock your knees), drop your neck gradually and let your trunk hang loose from the hips. Drop your shoulders and then your back as your arms and hands hang down. Do this two or three times until you feel completely relaxed. Then reach down as far as you comfortably can. If you have followed the full program, you should be able to touch the floor, or at least get a few inches closer than you would have before this exercise session.

Now gently work your way back to relaxer-cise number 1—and take the day off.

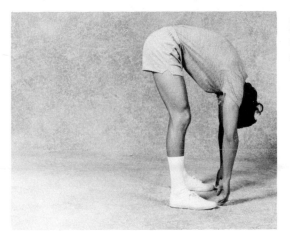

When a Disk "Slips"

Physicians and chiropractors generally agree that most backaches can be treated with physical therapy and exercise. Surgery should be a last resort; it's risky and doesn't always work. This is particularly true of a laminectomy, the operation to treat a "slipped disk." The problem occurs when an injured or aging disk springs a leak, allowing the pulpy core to ooze out and press on a nerve. The surgeon's aim is to scoop out the ruined disk. If the patient is young, a laminectomy nearly always succeeds. However, older people—fifty and up—who make up the bulk of patients, have a success rate of only 35 percent.

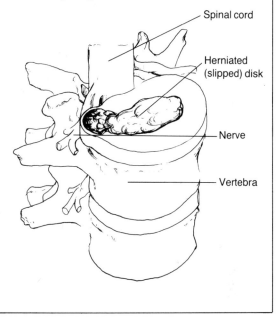

Spinal cord

Herniated (slipped) disk

Nerve

Vertebra

This completes the fit-back section of our back-relaxation kit. In the next chapter we'll continue with moves designed to soothe and amuse.

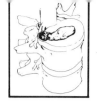

Chapter 9

Backsoothers
A Backlover's Guide

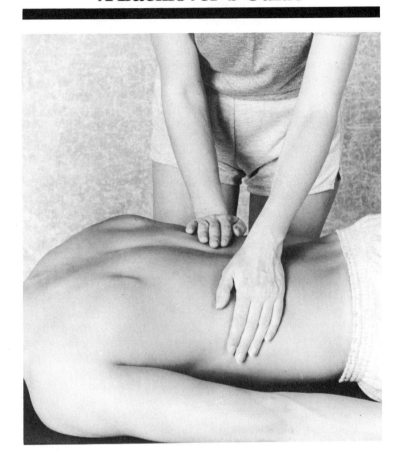

Back metaphors are telling: Carry the burdens of the world on your back; Put your back to it; Back him up. Of course, there's the "stout arm," but for the most part, the back—with its sturdy shoulders—is anatomy's less-than-perfect way of getting the job done. And as we've noted, mental stress can seep from cerebral circuits, tensing and tightening innocent back muscles.

Even well-trained muscles can get into trouble or may need protection from the daily crunch. And all backs enjoy pampering. A good back massage is one of the all-time great soothers—and not just for your back. In this chapter we'll start with a few emergency measures, in case you're already in trouble, and then go on to major and minor massages, other stretches, yoga moves, prevention, and a creative back-awareness routine.

EMERGENCY FIXES

Heat

 If you're immobilized by a painful back, heat, which increases blood circulation to the affected area, can help restore mobility.

Lie on your back, your head supported by a small pillow, your knees slightly bent and raised by another pillow. Put a heating pad or hot-water bottle under the painful spot. Apply heat for twenty to thirty minutes at a stretch, two or three times a day—but be careful not to burn yourself.

Ice

Though heat is the more common means of restoring blood flow to aching muscles, ice is useful for fast relief during the early stages of lower-back pain. But don't leave ice in any one spot for more than a few minutes lest it stop blood flow and cause muscle spasm.

Ice therapy works best when applied by someone else. If you find a kind soul who will help, have the person wrap some ice in a towel and stroke the skin on your lower back in steady sweeps from your buttocks to mid-back, about five minutes on each side. Place a small pillow under your stomach for support. No helper? Place an ice pack on your lower back—briefly.

MASSAGES

The Works

Whole-back massage, which requires a partner, is a great way to pleasure your back and relieve overall tension in your back and beyond. <u>Caution</u>: Although a massage is generally fine if your back hurts, don't try anything that seems to make it worse. Here are some general tips before you start:

■ Use a waist-high massage table if possible. It's easy on the massage giver's back and provides access from all sides. Next best is a firm, high bed. But the floor will do if you don't mind kneeling and bending over—and there's someone to massage you when you're done.

■ Massage oil makes the job easier. It reduces friction and makes the strokes flow more easily. Good commercial massage oils are available in health-food stores; pure almond oil and vegetable oils are popular products. Baby oil, if it doesn't contain mineral oil, is fine, too. When using oil, pour some on your hands first; then rub together to warm the oil.

■ One goal of a massage is to bring heat to the area. So keep the person warm and don't massage in a cold room. And—especially if it's a bit chilly—use a light blanket or sheet as a cover. Expose the area you're working on and cover it again as you move on.

■ The heavily muscled back can take more pressure than other parts of the body, but be careful to avoid pressing directly on the spine.

■ Don't massage any area that's infected: You may spread the infection or slow healing. And don't massage if there's a possibility of an injury, such as a broken bone, or if the massage seems to cause pain.

■ Be relaxed yourself when you give a massage, and pay full attention to what you are doing.

Here's a recipe for a basic massage:

1. Getting Started. Begin with a light, sweeping stroke down one side of the spine from neck to buttocks. Before one hand is done, send the other hand down the other side, overlapping strokes. If you're using oil, this motion spreads it over the whole surface.

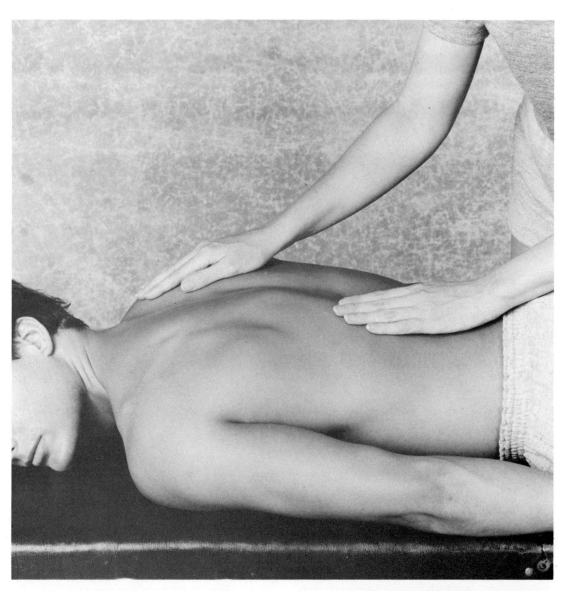

2. The Sweep Stroke. Place your hands on either side of the spine at the top of the back, with palm heels on the skin. Thumbs should point along the spine, fingers to the sides. Lean forward slightly and press down firmly with your own body weight, letting your hands slide down the length of the back. As your hands reach the hips, ease up, slide them out to the sides, and bring them back to the starting position—top of back, either side of the spine. Repeat several times.

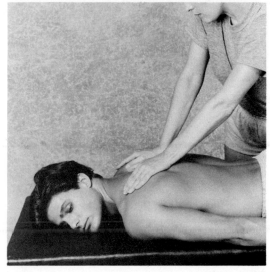

3. The Crisscross. Stand to the person's side and reach across the back with one hand; press the other hand against the near side. Using a heavy, even pressure, slide the hands toward the opposite side so they pass at the spine. Let up pressure as you cross the spine, but be firm over the muscles. Crisscross the entire back, top to bottom, with these strokes.

4. The Pummel. Open your hand; keep your fingers together. Now hold your hand vertically over the back, as if to deliver a karate chop. Now pummel or "tenderize" the major muscles in a light, rapid hacking motion, focusing on areas of pain or tension. Avoid the spine, bony areas, and the kidney region of the lower back. Sweep up and down each side or work on special areas of tension.

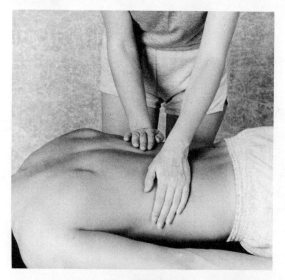

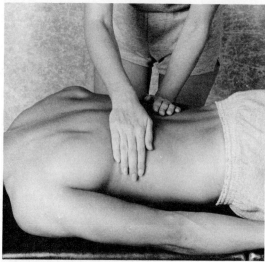

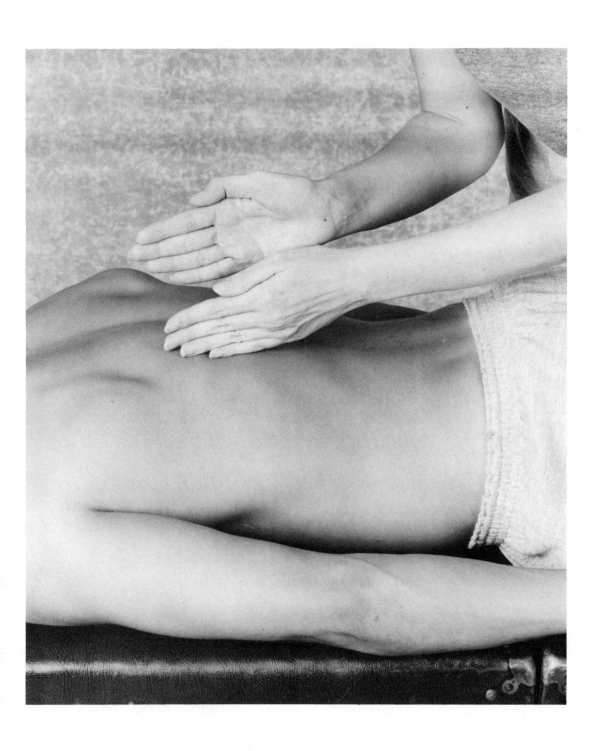

5. Trapezius Treat. The trapezius—the huge V-shaped muscle that wraps over your upper back and keeps your head in place—is a major tension collector. Everyone can use some help with this hardworking muscle. Here are some techniques:

Knead. Hold the muscle that runs from the neck to the shoulder between your thumb and finger, gently squeezing it as you knead it along its whole length from neck to shoulder. Repeat several times.

Knuckle. Make a fist, with your fingers touching the heel of your hand. Press down with the upper part of your finger (not the knucklebones) and use the flat surface to massage along the muscles you've just kneaded. Go back and forth from the shoulder up to the spine. Return to the shoulders with a lighter slide and repeat three or four times.

6. Lower Back. The latissimus dorsi, the large muscle running from the armpit to the lower back, is the villain in many cases of lower-back pain. Two strokes can relieve tension in this muscle or help stretch it so it will be less prone to spasm.

Stroke I. The first is a full-length stroke with your open hand, starting at the lower back. Keep your thumb extended and parallel to the spine, your fingers together at right angles to the thumb. Put your other hand on top of the first and with firm, steady pressure, slide both to the side. Use a lighter touch to slide back to the spine and move about half a hand upward on the back. Once you reach the shoulder blade, start on the other side.

Stroke II. The second stroke uses the forearm to sweep all the way up each side of the back in a single, wide movement. With fist clenched, place your forearm at the center of the back above the buttocks; use your other arm to hold your arm down in the middle. Use pressure from your forearm and hand as you sweep upward and outward toward the side— three or four times on each side.

For a finale, slide both hands slowly toward the neck and massage there with your fingertips for a few moments. Then slide along the shoulders and down the sides to the lower back. Stop and hold both hands there for a while. Then slide up to the shoulders, resting your hands briefly. Repeat three times, each time more lightly.

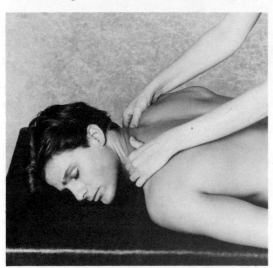

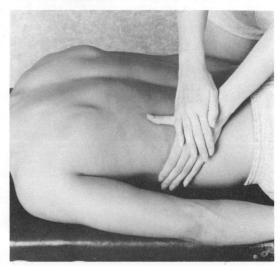

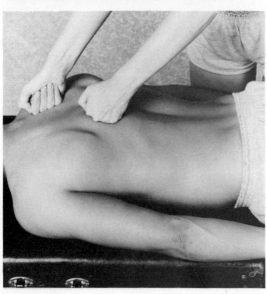

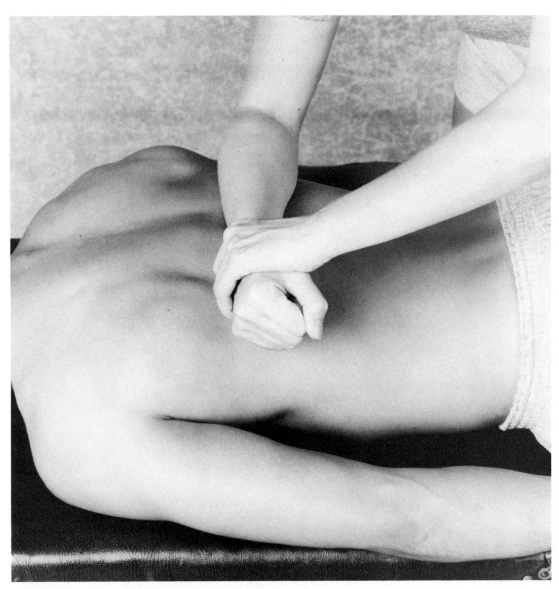

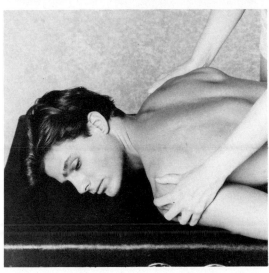

7. The Back Tickle. Here's a treat. It makes you feel relaxed as a kitten. The motion is a gentle back scratch using long, repetitive strokes. Using your fingers lightly, start at the base of the spine and stroke upward in a circular motion, or crisscross the back, side to side, or use long sweeps up and down. The key is a light touch in a repeated pattern. Continue for five minutes or as long as you want. Lovely, relaxing . . . zzzzzzz.

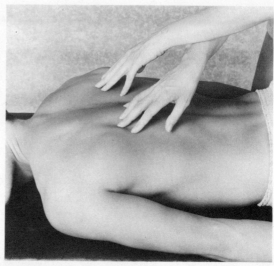

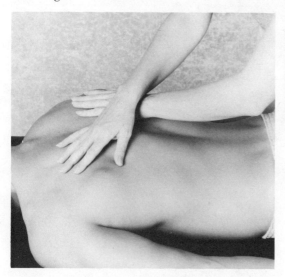

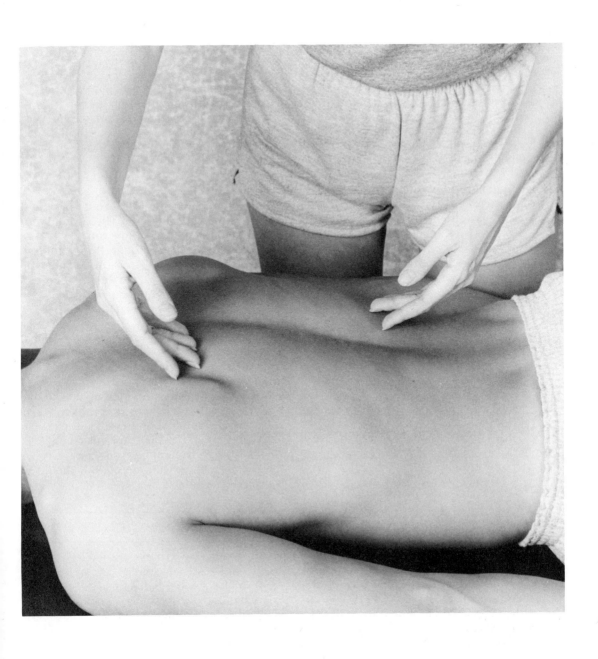

Do-It-Yourself Massage: The Jell-O Wobble

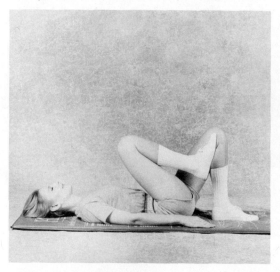 This exercise is useful as a quick fix for mild pain and tension buildup. Lie on your back, arms at your sides, legs stretched out comfortably. Scan your body from the back of your head, down your back, legs, and feet. Notice how your body touches the floor and note points of particular tension. Pay close attention so you can remember later how your back feels now.

Bend your knees and slowly slide your feet toward your buttocks. Feet are on the floor, about a shoulder width apart. Lift your right foot about six inches, so your knee is above your hip, and move your knee three to four inches toward your head, then back again. Repeat that movement—slowly at first, then increase the tempo. At the same time, make the movement smaller: faster and faster, smaller and smaller, so that it becomes a rapid jiggle.

Keep it up for a few minutes, letting yourself wobble like Jell-O. Now the other leg. Scan your back again. Better?

Do-It-Yourself Spot Massage

Thumb Massage

Sit upright, with your hands in the curve above your hips, your fingers along the side, and your thumbs at the back. Moving your thumbs in a circular motion, work up and down your lower back.

Lower Back

Lie on your right side and bring your right knee toward your chest. Reach around with your left hand as high up on your back as is comfortable. With your fingertips or thumb, massage firmly in small circles along the spine down toward the coccyx. Do three or four circuits up and back, and repeat on the opposite side. Don't strain—keep it comfortable.

Upper Back

Shoulder rubs are a good way to keep tension from building up during the day. Take a few minutes every half hour to give your shoulders a break. You can do this one at your desk. Reach your left arm behind your neck to touch your right shoulder. With your fingertips, massage as much of the trapezius triangle as you can reach, from along your spine next to the shoulder blade, and across the shoulder. Now the other side.

Rubber-Ball Massage

No massage partner available for those hard-to-reach spots? Try a firm but hollow rubber ball as a stand-in for the extra hands. Racquetballs, tennis balls, or handballs, even larger, spongy balls will work—experiment a bit. In a pinch, a pair of rolled socks will do.

Caution: Do not use balls directly on a painful spot; use them to get pressure to the points above and below the sore spots. Also, avoid direct pressure on the spine or near a disk or other spot that has given serious trouble in the past.

Do this massage either lying on your back on a firm surface or standing against a wall. Use two balls. To keep them in place, wrap them in a towel by twisting it at the center, putting a ball on either side of the twist, and then folding the towel closed at the ends. And if the towel is long enough, you can move your "masseuse" up and down by holding the ends of the towel.

Begin by placing the balls at the top of your back, on either side of the spine. To relieve tension in your shoulders, rest up to ten minutes with the balls pressing into your back. Relax your arms and shoulders, and each time you exhale, imagine your back muscles letting go—relaxing.

Reposition the balls a few inches lower on your back; spend a few minutes relieving tension there. Have a ball—continue down to the small of your back, spending extra time at tension-prone spots.

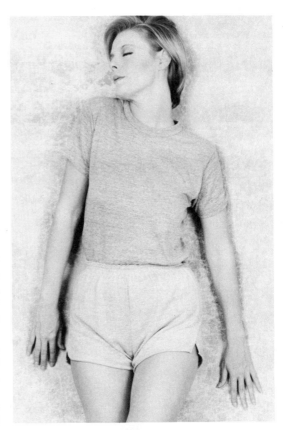

The Cat Wriggle

Cats do this one naturally. The idea is to use the weight of your body and easy, natural movements to massage your back. Try it lying down, sitting, or standing—in your office chair or while stuck in traffic.

If you're on your back, bend your knees, keeping your feet flat on the floor. Now wiggle your body from side to side, up and down. Move in any way that feels good.

If you're standing, find a friendly wall. Lean your back against it, your feet about a foot away from the wall. Let the wall support your weight while you roll side to side and wriggle around.

Hard but cushioned chairs work best for the seated version. Use your thigh and buttock muscles to lift your back up and down, rising slightly from the chair, then settling back into it. Let your shoulders lift up and down, but keep them relaxed.

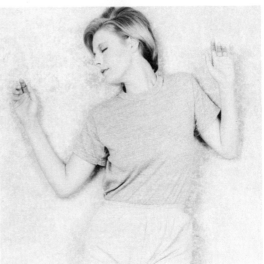

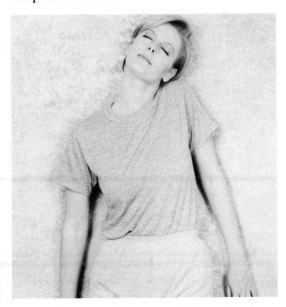

STRETCHES

Here are some useful stretches that will help cramped muscles relax. Try to work them into your daily routine.

Shoulder Rolls

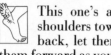 This one's a simple treat. Lift your shoulders toward your ears, draw them back, let them drop slowly, and move them forward as you come up again in a circular movement. Reverse direction. Sneak several of these in whenever you can.

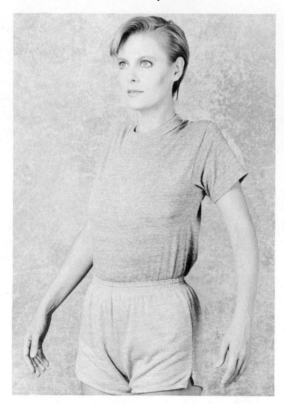

The Sink Stretch

Surprise—you're at the kitchen sink again! OK, make good use of it. Put your hands on the sink at arm's length, with your feet and shoulders aligned. (Use a sink, not a friend.) Bend your knees and tuck your bottom and head under, while your hips lean slightly backward. Now, making small movements side to side, stretch your bottom out behind you and slightly downward.

Inhale. Now exhale and let your back relax. Keep your lower back round as you stretch. Find the right pelvis tuck and knee bend to make this stretch feel right. S-t-r-e-t-c-h . . .

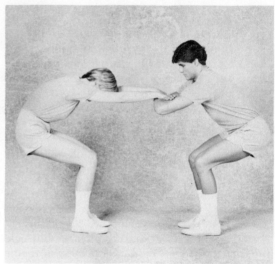

Stretch Workout

Groin Stretch

Lie on your back, knees bent, soles of your feet touching. Relax and let the weight of your legs gently stretch your groin muscles. Hold for about a minute.

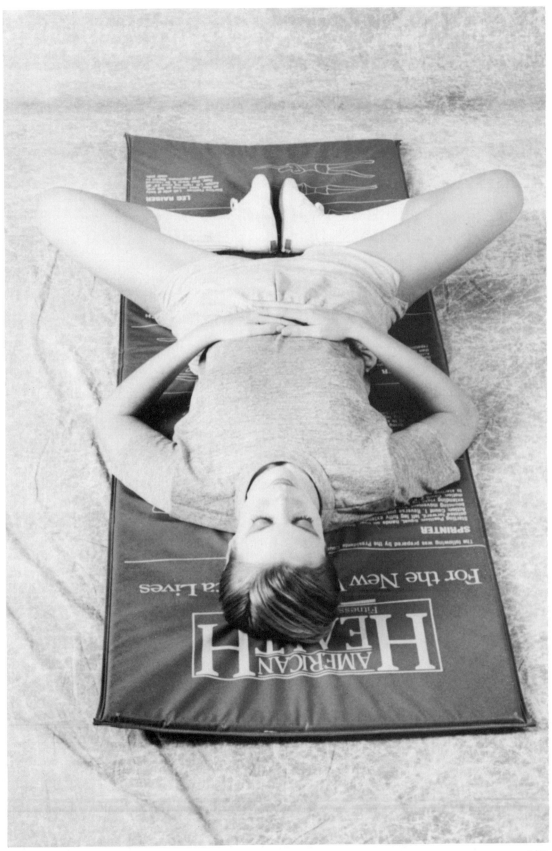

103

Neck Stretch

Now bring your knees together with your feet flat on the floor. Lock your hands behind your head and use your arms to gently pull your head forward. Stop when you feel a slight stretch through your upper back and neck. Hold for about ten seconds; then very slowly return your head to the floor. Repeat four to five times. Raise your head, pull it toward— but not up to—your knee on one side. Stop when you feel a gentle stretch through your neck. Then lower your head and do the other side. Repeat three times on each side.

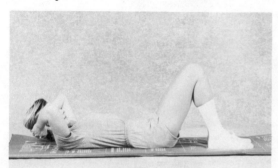

Side Stretch

With your knees still raised, stretch one arm (palm up) straight out above your head while the other arm (palm down) stretches down along your side. Stretch them in opposite directions, holding for eight to ten seconds. Repeat three times on each side.

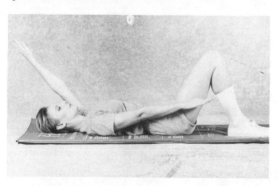

Total Stretch

Raise both hands above your head and stretch your legs down by pointing your toes. Reach as far as you can in both directions, holding for five to ten seconds. Then relax.

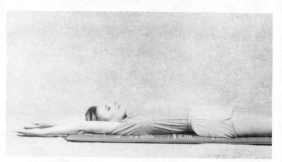

Fetal Roll

Pull both legs up to your chest, curling your head toward your knees. Grasp your knees with both hands and curl up. Feel the stretch in your upper and lower back.

Finale

Now go back to the total stretch, relaxing your whole body as you come out of it. Lie there for a few moments, letting your whole body go limp.

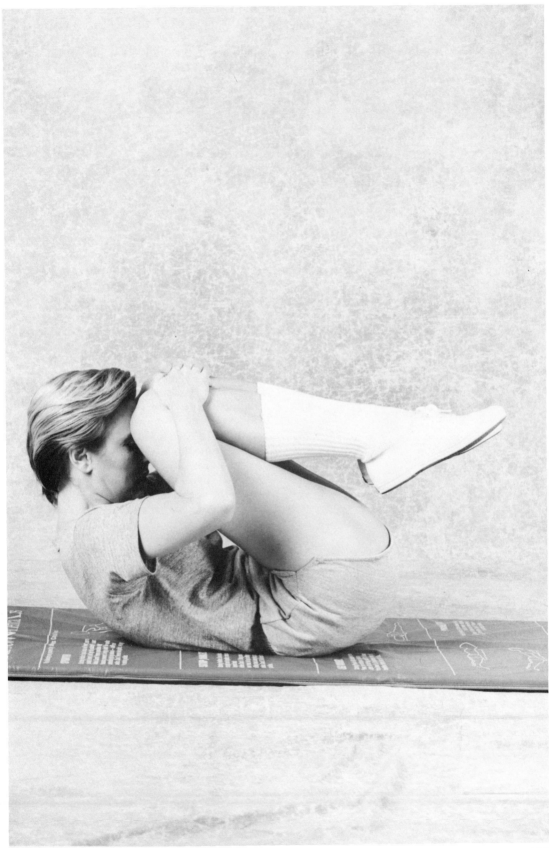

Yoga Moves

These are fairly traditional yoga postures—not just stretches. When doing yoga, the breath is often used either to bring your awareness to a particular area ("breathing into" it) or as an added relaxation measure. Yoga moves—with their emphasis on breathing—are another way of relieving stress and relaxing your back. Many people enjoy the physiologically pleasing combination of motion modulated by breathing. If the yoga approach interests you, see the Suggested Reading list, p.189, for more on this ancient discipline.

Yoga Breath I

Lying on your back, tuck your bottom so your lower back flattens against the floor. Exhale as you flatten your back, then release into the normal position as you inhale. Repeat six to ten times, breathing deeply and slowly.

Yoga Breath II

Now bring your right knee up toward your chest, hugging your leg as you exhale, releasing it back to the floor as you inhale. Repeat six to ten times, slowly. Now the left leg.

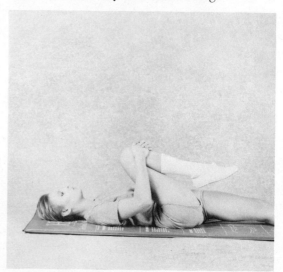

Lower-Back Twist

Lie on your back, arms out to your sides. Slowly bring your left knee toward your chest, inhaling as you draw it up. Exhale and gently lower your knees to the right side, twisting your pelvis as you do so. At the same time, turn your head to the left. Hold this position without straining for four to five deep, slow breaths. Then, on exhalation, untwist and return to the original position. Repeat on the opposite side. Doing this exercise daily will help keep your spine flexible.

REST POSITIONS TO SOOTHE BACK TENSION

Here's a good way to end a yoga session or relax after a stretching workout. If you have back pain, these gentle moves will help muscles relax.

Leg Hug

Lie on your back and hug both legs toward your chest. Hold as long as you like; it relieves pain or tension buildup.

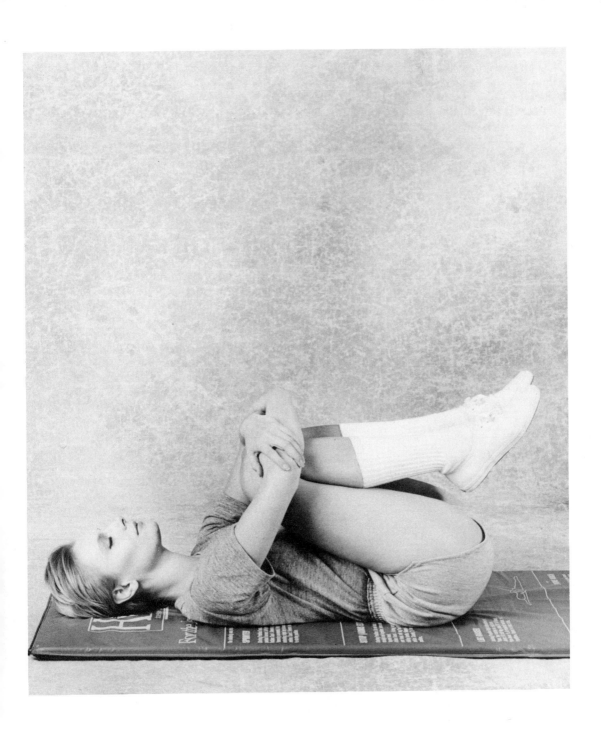

Lower-Back Rest

Lie on your back, knees bent, feet flat on the floor. Rest your arms on your chest or at your sides. Or put a pillow under your knees and let it bear the weight of your legs. These positions relieve lower-back tension.

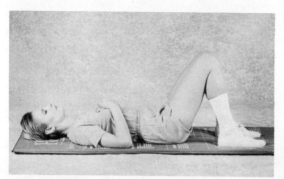

Baby Pose

Kneel and bend your upper body so it rests on your legs, your head gently touching the floor. Turn your head to one side and put your arms out above your head, or down to the sides. Now relax.

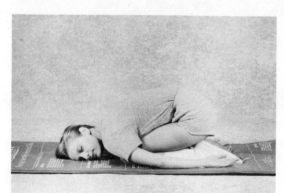

PREVENTION

About 80 percent of back pain, some say, is due to sedentary living and other afflictions of civilization. The less exercise you get, the more muscles strain to support your body and the more likely they are to accumulate tension. The desk job may well have created the current epidemic of back problems.

The best preventive measure is to pay more attention to how you use—and abuse—your back during normal routines, whether at work or at home. Throughout the day, tune in to your back's status as you sit, stand, walk, sleep. Even better, do a quick scan (see p.15). The time to intervene is at the first sign of tension buildup—not after the pain starts.

Think *back*. If you find yourself slumped over your desk or a keyboard, remind yourself to straighten your back and neck. Notice your posture from time to time—not with the tense inner admonition to "keep your back straight," but with a gentle reminder to ease up on those back muscles. Give them a break in the struggle against gravity by shifting to a more upright position.

Check in with your back regularly. If you feel a muscle starting to build tension, take a deep breath, then exhale and let the tension out. Drop your shoulders, too, and if you can reach the tense spot without straining, give yourself a minimassage.

Common Assaults

Sitting

Slumping, jutting your head forward, and chairs that don't fit right are common assaults on back tranquility. Sit well back in your chair so it bears your weight. Bend your knees slightly and keep your feet flat on the floor, your neck and head well supported and centered on your spine.

Lifting

You've heard it a hundred times, but it's worth repeating. Always flex your knees when bending to pick something up, and keep your back straight. Don't bend at the waist. If you're lifting something heavy, hold the object close to your body.

Weathering Winter

Cold weather contracts muscles and can aggravate back troubles. If you are prone to a particular neck or back knot, be sure to keep that area warm in wintery weather.

For more tips, see Chapter 15, "A New Look at Everyday Moves," p.173.

Sleep

Mattresses

The firmer the better. You will spend roughly a third of your life in bed. Do your back a favor and find a mattress that's firm but still comfortable. The average life of a mattress is ten years. If you're in the market for a new one, try it out in as many positions as you can, particularly your favorite sleeping curl-ups. Then go for firm. An "orthopedic" mattress may help if your back has been going into spasms and is especially stiff and achy in the morning. But that traditional remedy—a board under the mattress—may do just as well.

Backsoother Sleep Positions

It is best to sleep on your side, with a pillow under your head. The pillow should be neither too flat nor too high: The idea is to keep your spine and neck aligned.

If you are most comfortable on your back, put a pillow under your knees to help flatten your lower back, minimizing strain on those muscles—the chief hazard in that position.

And if it's got to be your stomach, put a small pillow under your hips to take pressure off your lower back. Extend your arm above your head on the side you are facing.

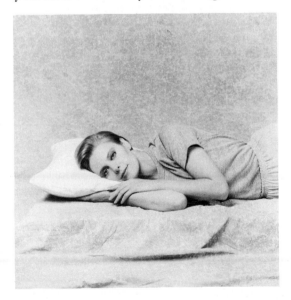

Getting Out of Bed When Your Back Is Killing You

If you've been in this situation, you know that even the simplest movement can be agony. Here's how to ease out of bed:

Still in bed, draw your knees toward your chest. With your knees at a right angle to your body, roll to the side. Keeping your knees and hips flexed, use your arms to prop yourself into a sitting position, your legs dangling over the side of the bed. Bend slowly so your center of gravity shifts over your knees and feet. Now stand up s-l-o-w-l-y to as erect a position as is comfortable. Proceed directly to the yoga breaths, p.106.

Feldenkrais Awareness Moves for the Lower Back

This long exercise is designed to increase your awareness of how your back moves. At the same time, these movements will develop flexibility and suppleness, enhancing your body sense of how back movements are coordinated with the rest of your body.

Go through these motions with gentle deliberateness. What counts here is not vigorous movement, but the attention you bring to the movements of your body. If anything hurts, be more gentle and make a smaller movement. As you move, sense exactly what's going on in your body. Breathe deep and easy.

The goal here is to be aware of the quality of moving, not to make a given number of repetitions. Tune in to the details of the motion—the subtle stretch of muscle, the twist of leg and back, the shifts of weight. If you lose focus on a sensation, pause for a few moments to reconnect. Then continue.

Avoid exertion and let gravity do the work. Rest between movements, letting yourself sense your body, your breath, the map of pressures where your back meets the floor. Be leisurely—read ahead or ask a friend to help you with the directions.

■ To begin, lie on the floor on your back. Use a firm but comfortable surface and wear loose-fitting clothes. Now become aware of your body as it touches the floor. Scan it to find the points of greatest pressure where your back touches the floor. Notice how your shoulders touch the floor, the bend at the small of the back, your pelvis. Do you feel tension there, or resistance?

■ Bend your knees so your feet are flat on the floor, feet and knees spread about as far apart as your shoulders. Rest your arms along your sides on the floor.

■ Gently lift your pelvis, arching your back in the air. Stretch up and then lower back down to the floor. As you move, scan your whole back—neck, shoulders, then down to your knees. Repeat this movement a few times, slowly, tuning in to the stretch of muscles, the play of tensions, as you move.

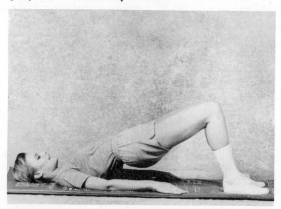

■ Bend your right knee only, bringing your right foot up till it is flat on the floor. Open your arms out level with your shoulders, your hands on the floor, palms up. Let your right knee drop over to the left by its own weight, letting your right foot turn out, though still in contact with the floor. Feel the points of tension in your leg and back. Then return your knee to the upright position.

■ Make this move several times, letting the weight of your knee do the moving. Notice carefully how your right hip rises, how the whole right side of your body is involved in the move, how the move affects your back and chest, and how your right heel rolls along the floor. Sense how your whole body is changed by the movement.

■ Breathe easily and deeply. Move very slowly, pausing at points along the way to sense how your body feels. Rest, bringing your arms and legs back down.

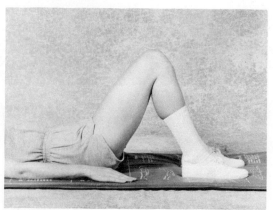

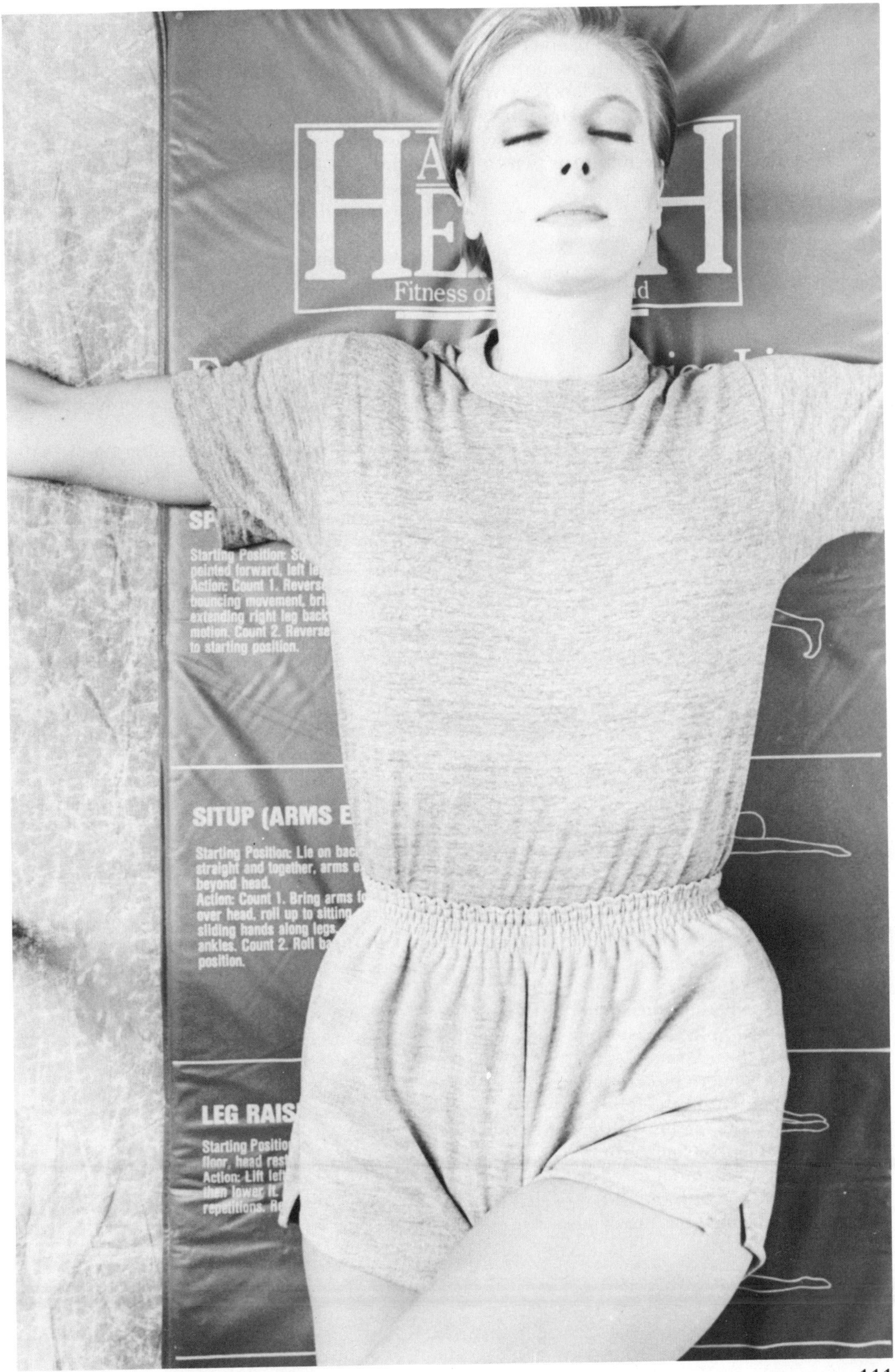
Fitness of
SITUP (ARMS
LEG RAIS
Starting Position: Lie on bac
straight and together, arms e
beyond head.
Action: Count 1. Bring arms f
over head, roll up to sitting
sliding hands along legs
ankles. Count 2. Roll ba
position.
to starting position.

■ Now expand the movement: Turn your head to the right as your knee bends over toward the left. As your head turns, notice the twist of your spine. Repeat slowly several times, enjoying the stretch. Each time you come back to center, sense how your pelvis presses against the floor as it returns to its natural position.

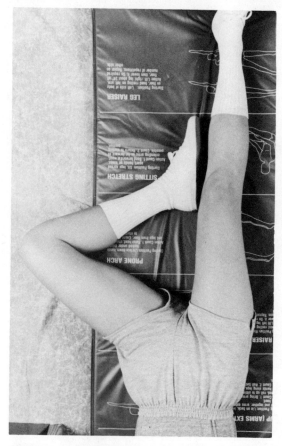

■ Bring your leg down flat, letting your arms find a comfortable position along your sides. Close your eyes for a few moments and scan your body. See whether you can notice the subtle way in which one side of your body feels different from the other.

■ Now bring your right knee up again, with your right foot flat on the floor. This time let the knee draw the leg out to the right, away from the other leg, so your right foot rolls to its outer edge. Without forcing, let the knee bring the leg down toward the floor of its own weight. Then bring it back to center.

■ Repeat the move several times, sensing the stretch and change through your body. Notice how, as your right leg moves out, your left leg rolls to the right, too. Feel the shift of movement through your back. Let your whole body assist with the movement, your chest lifting up slightly, your left hip rising, your spine twisting, your shoulders shifting. Notice all these coordinated shifts as you repeat the movement several times.

■ As you make these moves, let your left hip feel as though it is invited to join in the motion as part of the movement of the right leg. Sense how natural it is for the left hip to lift a bit from the floor each time your other knee moves right. Be sure your shoulders stay on the floor, so that your spine twists to accommodate the movement.

■ Now make the movement alternately to the left and to the right, from side to side. As your knee moves in one direction, let your head roll in the other. Pause for a moment at the end of each movement, your head pointing one way, your knee the other. Feel the way your whole body accommodates to the position. As you move back to center, notice how your body eases back to its natural position, as though you were being moved. Repeat on the other side—left knee up, right knee down.

■ With both knees up, leave the right knee upright as you move your left knee to the left side and back again. Move it to the left as far as you can without the right knee moving at all. Be slow and easy. Sense the pull in the right knee. Then let the right knee join in the motion of the swing to the left, as though it were being pulled along by the left knee. Let your knees come all the way to the floor on the left, and pause there, sensing your whole body. Do the same to the other side, the right knee leading the left. Rest, and scan your body.

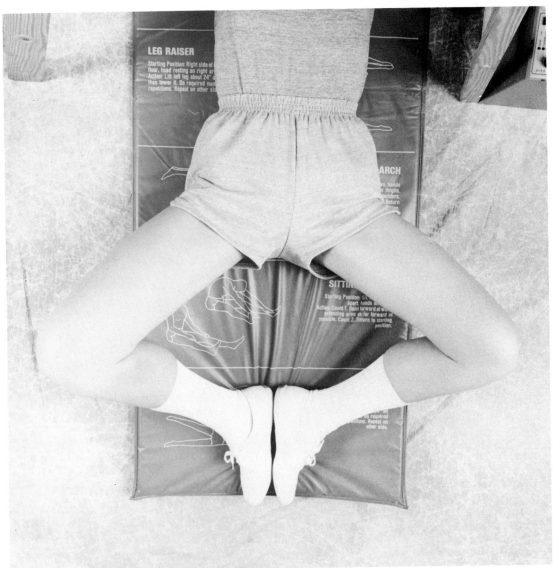

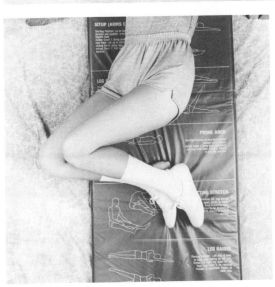

113

■ Next, swing both legs side to side a few times. Notice the changes in your lower back as the legs swing through their arc. Add to the motion by moving your head in the direction opposite to your knees. Again, tune in to the shifts throughout your back as you move, particularly the lower back.

■ Now slide your legs flat to the floor and rest, sensing how your body feels. Scan the pattern of pressure where your back meets the floor. Is more of your back touching the floor than when you began?

■ Arch your pelvis, just as you did at the beginning. Does it rise more easily? As you lie flat again, tune into your lower back. Is it flatter on the floor?

■ Rest for a few moments. When you feel ready, stand up slowly. Try to sense the changes in your back, legs, and shoulders as you stand and walk around.

These two back chapters have offered a smorgasbord of therapeutic moves. Help yourself to what makes sense for you, but keep in mind that a strong, fit back is the cornerstone of a relaxed body. Beyond that, try to be aware of what's happening to your back before it cries out in pain. Scan frequently to break the stress spiral. And even if it's generally well-behaved, don't forget that your large, muscled back may easily become a holding ground for tension that originates elsewhere.

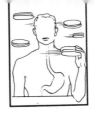

Chapter 10

Tension at the Dinner Table

The food may be fast,
but let the eater be slow.

Houseguests are coming, the car has expired, your boss needs everything yesterday, and the IRS has fingered you. . . . The bottom line: havoc in your digestive tract—nervous stomach, gastritis, heartburn, indigestion, belly bloat.

The digestive tract is an important stop on the tension trail. Like the heart, it's constructed largely of hardworking smooth muscle not directly under your control. At the same time, most of this system is a defenseless repository for stress. The stress may be mental—worry, tension, a harried schedule—or physical—gulping food or overeating. But the target is a physical system of muscle and hormone-secreting cells.

No doubt the stress of everyday living can tie knots in a delicate stomach, but until recently the care and feeding of the digestive tract was dictated by old wives' tales and medical misconceptions. Today physicians are abandoning old-fashioned dietary restrictions and stressing that *how* you eat may be as important as *what* you eat.

True, your digestive system may balk at certain foods, but the boring, rigid diets once prescribed have been jettisoned as useless—even harmful. It simply isn't true that food that burns your mouth will also burn your stomach; that hard-to-chew food is hard to digest; or that if your stomach acts up you need a "nursery diet"—soft, bland, pale-looking food.

Many digestive disorders respond to simple changes in diet and lifestyle. Food and tension are a bad mix. We now know that learning how to relax and taking steps to defuse a high-voltage schedule may help the dinner go down—and keep the medicine away.

To give your hardworking but vulnerable digestive system the tender, loving care it so badly needs, it's important to understand how each of its way stations functions. Let's begin at the mouth, where food is chewed and mixed with saliva, and follow it on a twelve-to-forty-eight-hour voyage down the digestive tract, marking the trouble spots. On the way, we'll find that a specific food may be the villain; other times tension and stress are to blame. And in certain cases—ulcers—we still can't pinpoint the cause.

ESOPHAGUS: HOME OF HEARTBURN

The esophagus is a narrow, foot-long muscular tube that contracts to push food along toward the stomach—even if you stand on your head. Esophagus and stomach are separated by an important valve—the lower esophageal sphincter. Contrary to general belief, heartburn is not a stomach disorder, but an inflammation of the esophagus. If its muscular lower sphincter leaks, acid gastric juice from the stomach bubbles up into the esophagus, causing a burning pain in the chest, usually low but sometimes as high as the throat.

About half of us suffer from heartburn, at least now and then. It is more common among overweight people and pregnant women. But because heartburn and a heart attack can cause pain in the middle or lower chest, telling them apart can mean the difference between life and death. For guidelines, see "Heartburn or Heart Attack?", p.118.

Because a full stomach puts extra pressure on the lower esophageal sphincter, overeating invites heartburn. But anything else that increases abdominal pressure may provoke backflow, so avoid tight clothing and don't bend forward or lift heavy objects soon after meals. Since gravity tends to keep stomach juices from backsliding, don't lie down for several hours after eating.

Since heartburn is caused by stomach acid, anything that washes away the irritating juices—a few swallows of water or food—will cure it. Antacids also help. But for more than temporary relief, simple dietary adjustments and relaxation are the key factors.

Not surprisingly, stress and heartburn go hand in hand. Tension may stimulate gastrin, a hormone that revs up the flow of acid gastric juices. Stress-related behavior—eating on the run, gobbling, midnight munching—means poorly chewed food, a cramped, overworked stomach, and increased abdominal pressure. Worse, two popular stress antidotes, alcohol and nicotine, further relax the sphincter to let stomach acid through.

The sphincter may also leak in response to certain chemical relaxers in fats, oils, chocolate, mints, and carbonated beverages, as well as personal food idiosyncrasies. Onions, peppers, lettuce, and spicy Mexican and Chinese food are common culprits. Once it's inflamed, the esophagus may become abnormally sensitive to spices, juices, and alcohol. Avoid them until symptoms disappear for a few weeks.

STOMACH: THE GRISTMILL

The stomach is a muscular bag that stores, crushes, and mixes food with water. You can live without a stomach entirely, but you'll suffer if you mistreat it. Since the stomach is essentially a food sack, ailments come in two basic varieties: pain when it's empty and pain when it's full.

When there's no localized disease, such as an ulcer, empty-stomach pain is called gastritis. It can be caused by excess acid, a sensitive stomach, or an irritant such as aspirin or alcohol. Its main symptom is burning or gnawing upper-abdominal pain at least an hour after a meal. If aspirin is the problem, take pills with food or a full glass of water. Avoid plain aspirin or try aspirin-free products such as acetaminophen or ibuprofen.

Other drugs—arthritis and asthma medications, antihypertensives, and antibiotics—may also be to blame. A note to the stress-prone: Nicotine and caffeine (as well as decaffeinated coffee) stimulate acid flow, and excess alcohol can inflame gastric tissues. Try to substitute a favorite relaxer—physical activity, progressive relaxation, meditation, the quick scan (if time is short)—for a drink or that extra cup of coffee. The roll-breathing exercise (p.120) may also help calm you down.

Symptoms of ulcers, the big-league acid disease, are so similar to gastritis that only X rays or a more specific test can tell the difference. Ulcers, which afflict 5 to 15 percent of the population, usually occur just beyond the stomach proper, in the duodenum, the first part of the small intestine. Whether it's gastritis or an ulcer, dietary treatment is the same: Cut out irritating drugs and foods, and neutralize the acid.

Since food neutralizes acid, a snack is a good remedy for the pain. So are antacids and prescription ulcer drugs such as cimetidine, which either cut antacid production or coat injured areas of the stomach. All of these therapies have about the same success rate: 85 to 90 percent after several months. But if treatment is stopped, up to 90 percent of ulcer sufferers will have a recurrence within six months.

DIET, STRESS, AND DOGMA

Hoping to speed healing, doctors once wedded science to myth and produced the old-fashioned ulcer diet. Milk and cream seemed soothing, so patients were told to drink up.

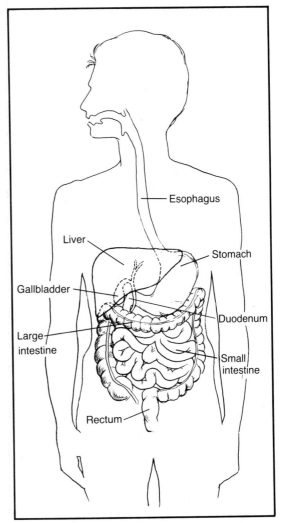

Seasoning and tasty foods were forbidden on the theory that arousing the taste buds must also stimulate the stomach. "Good" foods were bland: cooked cereal, rice, white bread, gelatin, cottage cheese, noodles, boiled eggs, and fish. These diets worked, but for a quite different reason. Since food relieves acid pain, patients ate and snacked more often. The ulcers healed—and the patients got fat.

But some doctors were uneasy. As far back as 1952, studies showed no difference in healing between patients sentenced to the boredom of an ulcer diet and those who ate whatever they wanted. Worse, scientists found that protein and calcium are acid *stimulators*. Since milk and many bland foods are rich in these nutrients, the diet could actually aggravate the ulcer.

Nowadays, doctors have walked away from the bland-diet myths: that tasteless foods are particularly soothing, and that white meat (allowed) is purer than red meat (forbidden). There's no proof that fried foods damage the stomach. Nor do sharp-edged foods—carrots, toast—cause irritation. Today's experts advise gastritis and ulcer sufferers to stay away from aspirin and arthritis drugs, plus alcohol, nicotine, and coffee. Period. In fact, smoking may be a major villain. A recent multicenter study indicts smoking as a major factor in slowing ulcer healing and causing recurrence.

But what about stress? The idea that stress is linked to ulcers goes back to the Greeks. Although stress may make an ulcer feel worse, the evidence that stress or suppressed anger *causes* ulcers is surprisingly weak. The overall incidence of ulcers reached a peak in the 1950s and then started to fall. It's unlikely anyone would claim the past thirty years have been increasingly tranquil.

Studies of people in stressful jobs find they do not have a higher risk of *developing* ulcers. And calm, relaxed people are as likely to get ulcers as hard-driving competitive types. One study of a high-stress group—air-traffic controllers—found an ulcer rate no different from that of the general population. Studies of twins suggest there may even be an inherited tendency to develop ulcers.

For now, the cause of ulcers continues to elude the experts. However, if you already have an ulcer, stress and tension may make it act up. And, of course, if stress causes a smoker to light up more often. . . .

If ulcers are your problem, the suggestions that follow at the end of this chapter may help you unwind body and mind.

BELLY BLOAT AND "NERVOUS STOMACH"

Pain on a full stomach usually comes from overload: If you suffer regularly, you may be overeating without realizing it. Or trying to cram too much into your day, you may be eating too fast, or swallowing air. To avoid the bloated pain of a stuffed stomach, cut back on

Heartburn or Heart Attack?

■ Heart pain is severe, usually "crushing" or "squeezing." Indigestion or heartburn is just that—"burning." Belching, nausea, or vomiting can accompany either.

■ Heart pain lasts. Call a doctor if two to four tablespoons of antacid doesn't help within fifteen minutes.

■ New or unusual pain should be checked out medically. Don't panic if you're low-risk: A heart attack is rare among men under thirty-five and women under forty. But after forty, think heart, not stomach.

large meals, slow down, and take care not to swallow air while you eat. Beans and other "gassy" foods are not responsible for air in the stomach, but carbonated beverages, beer, and whipped foods are big offenders.

If you eat modestly and chew well but still suffer pain, you may have a "nervous stomach." The stomach is a muscle; if tension makes it contract, it will be overloaded and you'll have a stomachache, just as tense back muscles produce backache.

The best cure for a nervous stomach is relaxation. If alcohol agrees with you, a single pre-dinner glass of wine deserves its long tradition as a digestive aid, particularly if accompanied by friendly small talk. Talking, resting, reading, even a brisk walk or other exercise before meals will make the stomach more receptive. If these measures don't help, try four or five smaller meals a day. Meditating, progressive relaxation, or autogenic suggestion (see Chapter 2, "Tension Targets," p.11) can also help you unwind, and the instructions on "mindful eating" at the end of this chapter should ease you out of a frenetic eating style. Of course, see your doctor to make sure nervous stomach is all you have.

ALL GALL

The gallbladder is often the source of digestive mischief, but, interestingly, it's *not* a tension target. The thumb-sized organ stores and concentrates bile, an oily substance produced by the liver. Bile flows through a duct into the small intestine, where it helps dissolve fats. The most acute digestive pain occurs when gallstones form, move out of the gallbladder, and block the duct carrying bile from the gallbladder to the small intestine. Fatty food is no longer blamed for gallstones. Passing a stone is simply a random event unrelated to diet—or stress.

Mindful Eating

Here's an exercise that may help you slow down. It's called mindful eating because these days food is all too often consumed by mindless eaters. How often have you gulped lunch at your desk, downed unnamed somethings while rushing about your house doing chores, or gobbled dinner against the family's pitched battles? Sad to say, eating is often one of those unconscious things we do on "automatic," like brushing our teeth.

But it's quite possible to eat with utter mindfulness, paying close attention to every bite. Food eaten with care is far more delicious than food eaten unnoticed; food eaten mindfully is well chewed and so more easily digested. Also, it's harder to overeat when you pay attention. Finally, to eat mindfully, you've got to get yourself into a calm, relaxed, and focused state of mind. That, for our purposes, may be the greatest benefit of all.

Mindful eating is simple. All you do is slow down, bring all your attention to what is actually happening while you eat—and keep it there. Obviously, this is is not an eating style to be followed literally in daily life, but it's a valuable exercise for harried, on-the-go eaters who want to get some control over mealtime. In Asia mindfulness of eating is actually taught as a form of meditation. Here's how:

Get some shelled nuts, corn chips, or anything you can eat in discrete units. Put them in front of you. Take a few minutes to become composed—take a slow, easy breath or two. Don't begin mindful eating until you are totally focused on what you're about to do.

Let's say you're going to eat almonds. Pick one up and hold it between your fingers. Pay careful attention to the exact sensation as the almond touches your fingers; feel the texture of its skin on your fingertips, the shape and pressure of holding it. Look at it: notice the grooves along its sides, its color and outline.

Now get ready to eat it, but do everything *very* slowly. Begin by slowly raising the almond to your mouth. Notice the moment you can first smell it—still several inches from your lips. If you're attentive, you may notice you've started salivating. Be aware of the first brush of the almond on your lip.

Next, put it in your mouth and start chewing, slowly and deliberately. Notice the feeling of your teeth biting through the almond and the work your tongue does moving the chunks of almond around your mouth. Note the nut's taste. Listen to the sounds of chewing. Tune in to the sensations created by every bite.

Notice how the chewed almond bits mix with saliva as you swallow. And be sure to chew all the bits completely and to swallow them *before* you take another bite. Continue eating the almond—and all the rest—with the same careful deliberateness. Stay calm and focused through it all.

This mindful mode of eating can be adapted to any meal if you remember to stop, calm down, and pay attention to your food. If you suddenly catch yourself racing mindlessly through yet another meal, just slow down and take a few mindful bites.

THE SMALL INTESTINE: HEAVY-DUTY DIGESTION

The twenty-foot-long small intestine is the workhorse digestive organ. Here food is bathed in digestive juices and broken down into simpler nutrients, to be absorbed into the blood. You can live without the other digestive organs, but not without the small bowel.

Fats are not digested until they reach the small intestine, and here they cause little trouble, despite the persistent belief that fried or greasy foods are hard to handle. Naturally, it's sensible to avoid any food that upsets you, but there's no evidence the human body has more difficulty with fats than with proteins or carbohydrates. Curtailing fats may be important for weight loss or preventing heart disease, but no common digestive problem requires a low-fat diet.

Ironically, you may suffer real digestive mischief from innocent-sounding milk. Most babies digest it easily, but as we mature, many of us stop manufacturing lactase, the small-intestine enzyme that breaks down lactose (milk sugar). Thus, it pours from the small intestine into the large intestine where bacteria ferment it: Gas, cramps, and diarrhea are the result. Before you blame repeated bouts of such misery on your boss or loved ones, make certain milk products are not the villain.

And if you have a flatulence, or gas, problem, it's probably your diet rather than stress that's to blame. Complex carbohydrates found in beans, whole grains, cabbage, and fruits such as prunes and grapes pass largely undigested through the small intestine to the large intestine or colon, where resident bacteria break them down. Unfortunately, colon gas may be a by-product. To prevent gas, avoid troublesome foods.

119

What Causes the "Butterflies"?

A deadline is closing in on you; you're about to make a speech, take an exam, or go to a job interview. You've got the jitters in your head and "butterflies" in your stomach. That tight, quivery feeling in the pit of an uneasy stomach is not a digestive disorder but a mixture of muscle tensions. The rectus abdominis, the long, flat muscle running up the abdomen from the pubis to the ribs, tenses, causing the jittery sensation; the stomach muscles themselves may contract, producing the tight, constricted feeling.

To help banish butterflies, use a few deep, calming breaths. First inhale and then as you exhale, let the tension drain out of your body . . . out of your neck, shoulders, back, abdomen. Feel your hands and legs go flop. Shake them; now breathe in and out again . . . once more. Better?

Any of the overall relaxation techniques in this book will be useful in extinguishing the jitters. If you have a partner, you may wish to try the following simple exercise.

Roll Breathing

Lie on your back. Have your partner put one hand on your abdomen and one hand on your chest. You will inhale and exhale as in deep breathing, but each in-breath is taken in two stages—abdomen, then chest. Imagine that you are breathing into your partner's hand as you fill your belly with air. When your abdomen feels full, continue breathing into your chest. Watch your hand as it rises. Then exhale fully through chest and belly simultaneously. Repeat. It's important to keep a rhythmic rolling effect between abdomen and chest. But breathe at your natural pace.

Breathing while concentrating on the belly induces relaxation; chest breathing seems to increase energy. Thus, this exercise is both energizing and relaxing.

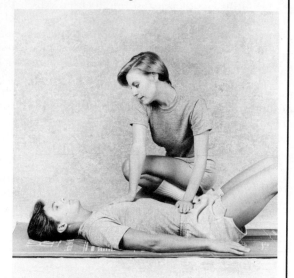

THE LARGE INTESTINE: STORAGE

Attached to the small intestine in the right lower abdomen is the large intestine or colon. A muscular tube the diameter of your fist, its job is to process and *store* undigested food. Many people believe the colon's job is "to get rid of waste." This is a poor description, leading to an unwholesome concern with bowel movements.

The colon needs plenty of indigestible residue (fiber) to function properly. If there's not enough residue, the bowel may ignore it, leading to constipation. If the bowel tries to move a small pellet of waste along, it must squeeze down to pencil size to get behind and push. Excessive contraction causes cramps. What's more, a big muscle pushing a tiny load can move it too rapidly. Result: diarrhea. These complaints—irritable colon—account for 60 percent of the patients gastroenterologists see.

The lack of fiber in the standard U.S. diet is probably responsible for the prevalence of irritable colon, although stress may aggravate the condition. At one time, the "residue" left after digestion was scorned as a nonfood and considered the source of dangerous "toxins." Today fiber, the indigestible matter in fruits, vegetables, and whole grains, has become a nutritional hero. It provides the colon with waste matter to store until there is sufficient bulk to be moved along without exaggerated colon contractions.

For this reason the colon works best if allowed to do its job—store waste. It will empty sooner or later; there's no need to get uptight about hurrying the process. If you were born with a three-times-a-week bowel, nothing will convert it to a daily schedule. If constipation is a problem, above all, try to relax about the bathroom scene and avoid "toilet stress." Instead, try vigorous exercise or a brisk walk, followed by a hearty breakfast, including coffee and a large glass of juice. The slight dehydration caused by exercise combined with fluid and coffee, a bowel stimulant, is an unstressful way of awakening a sluggish bowel.

Medicine has come a long way in revamping guidelines for healthy digestion. Complicated, rigid diets are out. Today the experts recommend omitting only those foods you know cause problems. Above all, relax—eat less, eat slowly, eat pleasantly. Even the fast-food counter can be tamed: Let the food be fast, but the eater slow.

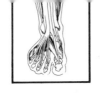

Chapter 11

Pampered Feet

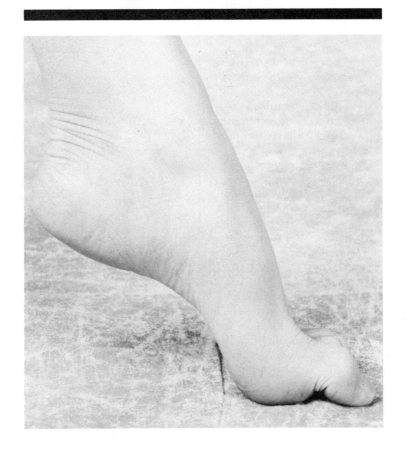

When it comes to the lowly foot, we deal with stress in its most straightforward physical sense. A complex jigsaw of 26 bones, 19 muscles, and over 100 ligaments and 31 tendons, the foot is an engineering marvel that combines the best features of beanbag, lever, and concrete.

Its durability is remarkable. You average 8,000 to 10,000 steps a day, which adds up to 115,000 miles in a lifetime. With each step, your foot carries 120 percent of your body weight—two to three times your weight when running. If you weigh 150 pounds, your foot braces about 125 tons of force for every mile you walk. That's stress!

Except when you kick off your shoes and collapse in agony at night, relaxation doesn't seem to be the foot's lot in life—unless you help out. Furthermore, your feet are at an additional disadvantage. They are at the greatest distance from the heart and so are prone to blood-flow problems, both coming and going. This makes them especially vulnerable to muscle knots and cramps and perfect candidates for soothers, like massage, that stimulate blood circulation.

Eighteen of the foot's muscles are on the underside, where they spread, support, and curl the toes; some support the arch. The nineteenth muscle, on the top, splays to help lift the toes. Twelve other muscles, originating in the lower leg, extend through to the foot, where they help control movement and maintain balance. For example, some muscles in the front help you point your toes.

Because the foot and legs are so intimately connected, a problem in one place can affect the other. A pain in the top of the foot, for example, may be due to tension in the lower leg. And cramped arches can mean tension in the calf. The foot-leg connection also applies to blood flow. Leg tension can lead to poor foot circulation and muscle cramps.

Alas, poor feet. Meant to be footloose and free to receive the earth's massage, they're imprisoned in tight shoes, then ignored and abused. They deserve better. The relaxed, awakened foot is a sensual delight. Pamper them, soothe them—then put your best feet forward.

MASSAGE

There are many foot-massage techniques; feet, after all, are easy to reach. To start, wash and dry your feet, and have skin cream or massage oil handy. Many people find that a foot massage leaves them relaxed all over.

Caution: If you have phlebitis or thrombosis, a foot massage could dislodge clots. Be careful if you have varicose veins or are recovering from a fracture—check with your doctor first. Also avoid foot massage if you have a fever or an infection lest the infection spread to other areas.

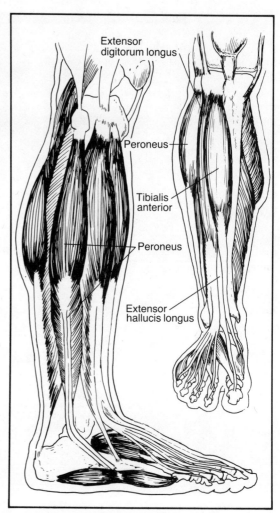

Shiatsu and Reflexology

The Oriental technique shiatsu—or in modified version "reflexology"—traces a map of all the body organs on the sole of the foot. The ancient belief is that the foot has nerve endings that lead to these organs, and that by massaging the appropriate regions on the sole of the foot and the toes, you can heal problems elsewhere in the body.

Though there's nothing in modern physiology to support the claims of reflexology, a thorough foot massage can leave you feeling so relaxed and refreshed, you may almost believe it's true.

The shiatsu basic stroke is steady pressure—for about three seconds—produced by the ball of the thumb. For easy access to the foot you are working on, sit with it resting on the opposite knee.

Begin by grasping your big toe between your thumb and index finger, the thumb on top. Press for about three seconds, release, and move to another point to press again. Move to the other toes.

Spend some time on the top of your foot, pressing along the web of tendons that run to each toe and out along the toe as you did with the big toe.

Now spend a good deal of time going over the whole surface of the sole, front to back, side to side, in a series of presses and squeezes. Move on to the next sector after each squeeze. Cover the entire sole; then head up the sides about ankle-high. Find the spots that feel best for you and spend more time working on them.

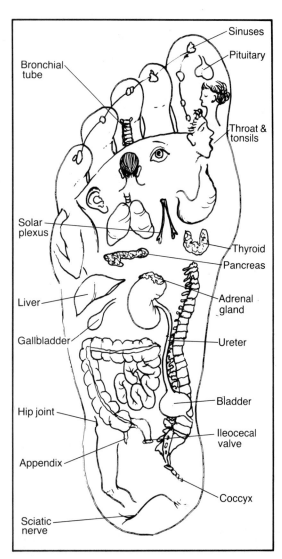

Whole-Foot Massage—For Yourself

The stroke that works best is a circular motion using the firm pressure of your thumbs or strongest fingertips.

Deep Massage
Grip the foot between your hands, with fingers on the sole and thumbs on the top. Work the bones deep inside the foot by pressing outward with the heel of each hand and up and in with your fingers. Then rotate the bones by moving one hand up while the other moves down. Work the length of the foot. Be firm.

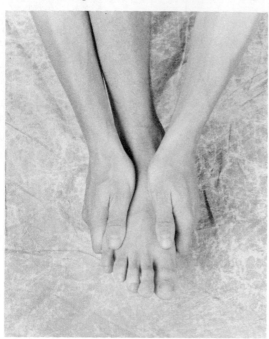

Quick Massage
Using your fist, work oil or cream into the sole of your foot. Work in circles from top to bottom. Now hold the top of the foot with your fingers and knead the sole with your thumbs. Next, use all your fingers to work the heel and around the ankle. Finally, tug each toe.

Golf Ball. If you don't have time for this routine, just roll a golf ball around under the sole and arch of each foot, then up and down the sole. Press as hard as feels good.

Knuckle Arcs. Make a fist with one hand and hold your foot with the other. Massage the sole with your knuckles, moving in small circles from toe to heel.

Thumb Press
Hold your foot with your thumb on the sole and fingers on top. Press in hard, firm circles over every patch of the sole. Then do the same over the top of the foot. Be thorough. Use your fingers to press near the ankle and heel.

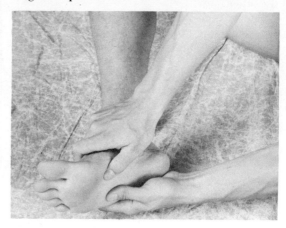

Massage Stretches for Toes

Hold the heel with one hand. With the other, push the toes forward and back. Hold the stretch for a few seconds each way. Repeat.

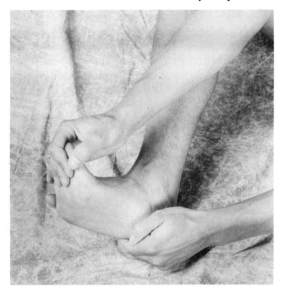

Slap

It's a long way from heart to foot, and blood circulation may be sluggish at this distant outpost. Brisk slapping can stimulate circulation and invigorate a weary foot. With one hand, grasp the foot under the ankle. With the other, slap the bottom, top, and sides of the foot.

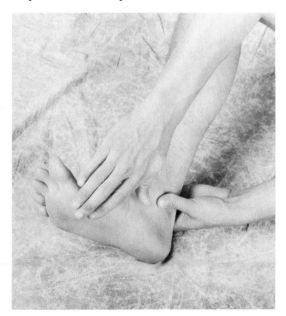

Toe Tugs

Gently tug each toe, one at a time, with your index finger and thumb. Then, starting with the big toe, twist from side to side like a corkscrew, letting your thumb and forefinger slide off the end. But don't crack the toe knuckles.

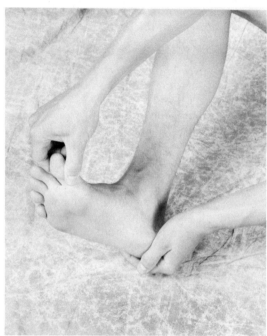

Whole-Foot Massage—For a Friend

A good foot massage is one of the nicest favors you can do a friend. Have your friend lie faceup so you can face the sole of the foot. Hold the foot with the fingers of both hands on the sole, thumbs on top.

Work the sole of the foot, applying pressure with your fingers, massaging up and down the sole.

Spend special time on each toe, massaging it between your thumb and forefinger. End by giving it a gentle tug.

Work around the ankle with your thumbs, spending more time in the area under and around the anklebone.

Using the pad of your thumb, stroke along the tendons that lead to the toes, moving from the large to the small toes.

Now make a fist; steady the foot with your other hand. Massage throughout the sole with your knuckles. Move in small circles, pressing firmly, from the heel to the bottom of the toes.

To finish, hold the foot between your hands, one palm on the sole, the other on top. Hold the foot a moment—then sweep down from the ankle to the toe tips.

Caution: Many people have very sensitive feet. If you hit a ticklish or sensitive spot, be careful. The idea is relaxation—not to produce more tension.

STRETCHES

The muscles in your feet and lower legs love a good stretch. Here are some stretches you can do whenever you get a free moment. Just slip off your shoes and alternately tap the floor with your heels and toes. Feel the stretch in your calf muscles and the Achilles tendon at the back of the foot. Then rotate your feet; fan out the toes. Wake those muscles up!

Ankle Stretch
Hold your foot with one hand under the heel. With the other, gradually push the top of the foot away from you. Hold the stretch, then pull the top of the foot toward you to stretch the top of the ankle. Repeat.

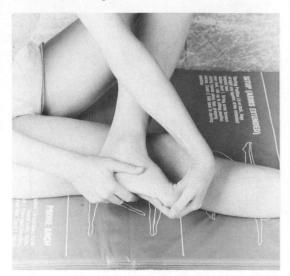

Toes and Arches
Sit on your knees with your toes underneath you. Lean forward on your hands, then slowly push back till you feel a comfortable toe and arch stretch. Hold for fifteen seconds.

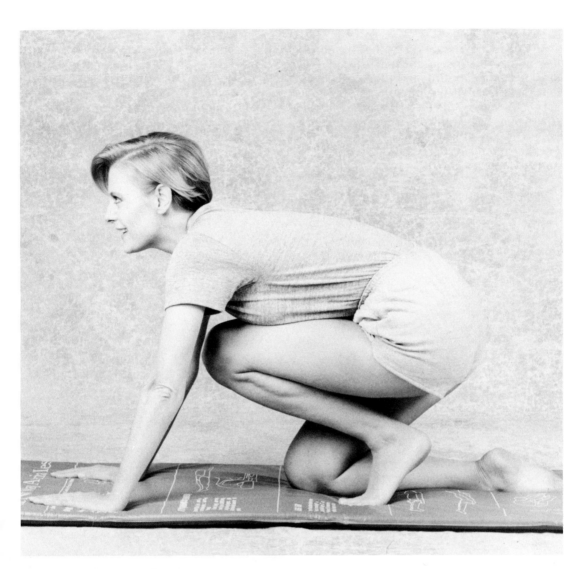

Ankles and Achilles Tendons
Sit on your heels with your toes flat. Bring one knee up to your chest, using your arms to help bear your weight. Lift the same heel about half an inch off the floor, then lower it as you push your shoulder and chest forward on the thigh. Don't try to get your heel flat. Gently stretch the Achilles tendon. Hold fifteen seconds and switch.

Inchworm

With one foot, press down the tips of all five toes, arching the area just behind to lift the ball of your foot and pull the heel forward (don't make a toe fist). Then with the heel in the same position, extend your toes to flatten the foot once again. Repeat till you've inched forward four to six inches. Then reverse: With your toes pressing and the rest of the foot raised, slowly pull your foot back to the start.

Total Foot Flex

Lie on your back, your feet apart. Flex your toes upward so you feel a stretch at the Achilles tendon. Hold for ten to fifteen seconds.

Next, point your toes inward, then outward. Hold each position ten to fifteen seconds. Finally, rotate your feet in ankle circles, four times in each direction. End by shaking your feet. Repeat the sequence five times.

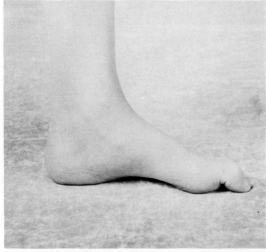

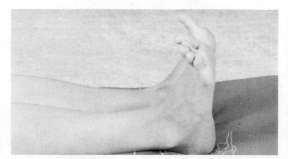

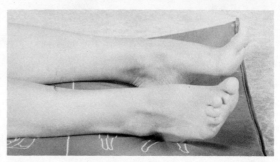

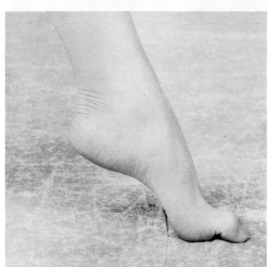

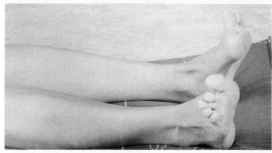

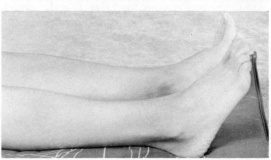

Toe Tricks

Sit on the floor so you can easily reach your bare feet. Keep your foot flat on the floor but flex your toes up from the floor. Now, one toe at a time, if you can, try to curl them back down, from your little toe to the big one. Three times for each foot.

Note: The little toe may be the most underused human appendage. If it lies there limp, help it along with your hand. At best, try to get some sensation into it.

Towel Challenge

Sitting or standing, place your foot on top of a towel on the floor. Spread your toes and grab the towel with them so you can pull it along the floor. Get your arch into the action. Don't move the towel with your heel—that's cheating. It may take a while before you can do this; these muscles have been hibernating inside your shoes for years.

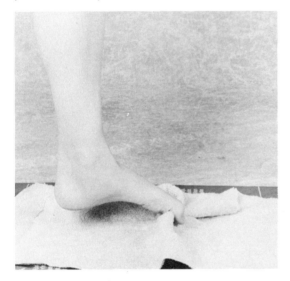

AWARENESS—MINDFUL WALKING

It's all too easy to forget about your feet—far away and hidden in shoes. But increasing awareness can pay off. Remember the eating meditation exercise, "Mindful Eating," in Chapter 10, p.119? Here's a walking meditation routine, "Mindful Walking," that shows you how to be focused even while active. This exercise not only increases foot awareness, but is great relaxation therapy because, like any form of meditation, it channels the mind and blocks out all other strands of mental activity. Here's how to do it:

Take your shoes off. Standing in one place, feel the sensations in your feet as they touch the ground. Stay with whatever you feel at each moment. As you are about to take a step forward, notice your mental intention to step forward. Slowly lift your foot, feeling every sensation—lightness, suspension, tension, motion—whatever feelings are present.

It's best to start at a slow pace so you can pay attention to the sensations. Eventually, you'll be able to go faster and yet maintain awareness. Move your foot forward, place it on the ground again, and shift your weight onto it. All the time, be aware of the sensations in this movement. When thoughts arise, don't be concerned with their content. Bring your mind back to your foot feelings and stay with this simple experience of walking. Continue to do this as long as you like—five minutes to half an hour or longer.

At first, to keep your mind focused, it helps to label the action. For example, you can say silently, "Up—forward—down," noticing the feeling of weight as it shifts from one foot to the other. Later you can simplify the process by eliminating the words. Just concentrate on the sensation.

To observe the process of mind in greater detail, note the intention that precedes each motion, as well as the sensations themselves. Thus: *intending* to lift, lifting; *intending* to move forward, moving forward; *intending* to place, placing; *intending* to shift, shifting.

Finally, you can develop a direct perception of the entire routine—intent, movement, sensations—without labeling any of it.

FOOT CARE

Here are some special tips and sensual treats for pampered, relaxed feet.

■ If, from time to time, you have to stand for hours at a stretch, try standing on the outer edges of your feet to reduce stress on the usual weight-bearing points.

■ Tired feet? Elevate them, preferably above heart level. Blood tends to pool in your feet. Raising them helps restore circulation.

■ Avoid ill-fitting shoes no matter how fashionable. Feet love low heels, ample toe room, and good arch support.

■ Be creative. Use feet instead of hands to turn the TV dial, pick up marbles, open a drawer. Take your shoes off at work and rotate and flex your feet back to life. Drop a pencil on the floor; pick it up with your feet.

■ Active feet are happy feet. Go barefoot when you can. But protect your feet from sharp, craggy surfaces or during rough sports. Shoes were invented for a reason.

■ Try a pedicure. (1) Soak feet for a few minutes in warm water. Dry and lightly powder them. (2) Smooth calluses and slough off dead skin with a wet pumice stone. Use a pedicure file to finish the job. (3) Cut the nails straight across. Soften cuticles with warm oil, then push them back. Now, if you wish, treat them to a massage. (See "Whole-Foot Massage— For Yourself," p.126.)

Foot Fun

You'll need a friend for this. Lie on the floor, the soles of your bare feet touching each other's. Use your feet expressively: Introduce yourself and tell something about yourself with your feet. Have a little foot fight, make up. Hug your partner's feet. Do something that feels good. Have fun.

As your busy life ticks around the clock, foot care may seem an afterthought, even a luxury. "I'll relax the rest of me," you say. "Feet can fend for themselves." A mistake. A good foot massage can spread its relaxed blessings to the rest of your body as well. And the time you take to cream, massage—even to do a desk-stretch routine—provides a brief oasis of relaxation in your day.

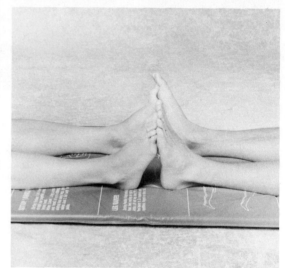

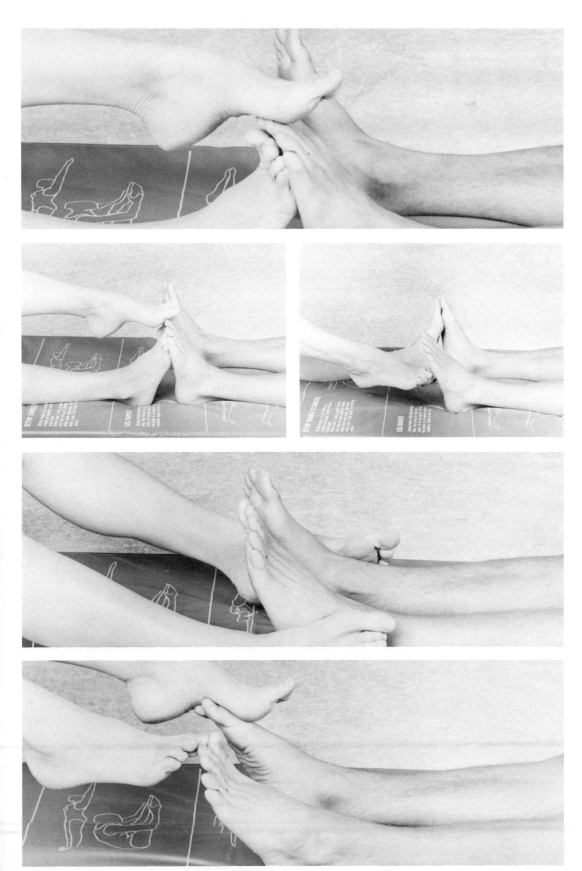

Part III: Night and Day
Chapter 12

Stress in the Bedroom

"A few minutes of peace
and quiet can be worth
four hours of foreplay."

Sexual passion is like a garden; it must be nurtured. But the demands of modern life can sap precious time and energy, so that on-the-go couples often find themselves too busy for lovemaking. And as a regular paycheck becomes a priority for women as well as men, often neither one has the emotional energy needed to tend the relationship—a job once assumed to be primarily the woman's.

Stress turns up regularly as the villain in a long list of unhealthy scenarios. Its impact on our sex lives, however, has been largely ignored. Yet when stress—from major crises to daily hassles—intrudes on a couple's private life, sexual response, frequency, and satisfaction may suffer. Although a stress-blighted sex life has mental origins, the physiological functions that make sexual response possible are highly sensitive to both emotional stress and physical exhaustion. In this chapter we will suggest ways to deal with the day's tensions and cultivate that relaxed, yet focused frame of mind so important for sexual pleasure.

From clinical cases sex therapists know that nonsexual pressures can puncture passion faster than you can say "Masters and Johnson." Warning signals may be a vague feeling that sex is more trouble than it's worth, a loss of sexual desire, and decreased arousal during sex. A person who can't switch mental gears from the role of jobholder, student, or parent to that of lover may not even notice a partner's caress. The distractions produce something like "highway hypnosis," but few people function well sexually on automatic pilot.

Consider George and Diane, a married couple in their mid-thirties with two children. They love each other and have no sexual hang-ups. Yet in the past few months their once-gratifying sex life has fizzled, sabotaged by stress.

A career couple, George and Diane are on the go from morning till night: working out before breakfast, getting the children off to school, battling commuter traffic, and juggling work problems; after work, the cleaner's, supermarket, dinner, pets, laundry, and the kids' homework. Weekends are a whirl of family, friends, shopping, and entertaining. By the time the frenetic duo crawl into bed, they are usually too tense and exhausted for romance. When they do make love, George may have trouble getting an erection; Diane's still making "to do" lists.

Aging and familiarity, of course, put some brakes on passion. But in their landmark study *American Couples*, sociologists Philip Blumstein and Pepper Schwartz also cite lack of time and energy as important reasons for the falloff. After you have read this chapter, you and your partner may wish to run through the checklist on p.140 to see whether stress is eroding your sex life.

THE PHYSIOLOGY OF AROUSAL

Severe stress not only overloads the mind, it may also short-circuit sex physically by upsetting the delicate neural choreography of the parasympathetic and sympathetic nervous systems. The sympathetic system mobilizes the body for action, making the heart pound, pupils widen, face flush, and skin perspire. In contrast, the parasympathetic system conserves energy and keeps all systems functioning at a steady, regular pace.

But timing is everything. During the early stages of sexual arousal, the parasympathetic system predominates. It relaxes the walls of arteries in the pelvic area, so that they dilate and blood flows in faster than it flows out. In men increased blood volume produces an erection; in women, it causes vaginal lubrication and swelling of the vulva, clitoris, and vaginal walls. This genital engorgement also contributes to the subjective feeling of arousal, though subjective and physiological responses don't always jibe.

Then as excitement mounts, the sympathetic system takes over. It pushes up the pulse rate, speeds breathing, tenses muscles—reactions that contribute to a feeling of sexual urgency and culminate in the muscular contractions of orgasm and ejaculation.

Strong emotions, including those linked to physical or psychological stress, can upset the critical balance, switching on the sympathetic system prematurely. Physical tension in itself is not the culprit; like laughter, sex first builds up tension, then explosively releases it. But problems can arise when sympathetic arousal turns on before blood-flow changes have prepared the way. (Interestingly, not everyone responds to stress with a loss of sex drive; sometimes a surge of adrenaline and increased muscle tension may increase erotic feelings.)

Stress may also interfere hormonally with sexual responses. Severe stress, such as soldiers experience in battle, lowers testosterone levels. The precise sexual role of testosterone—produced in the testes, ovaries, and adrenals—is not clear, but some researchers believe it must reach a minimum blood level for men and women to respond sexually.

Though some people turn to the bottle to solve the stress-sex problem, it is no solution. A glass of wine or a single drink can reduce anxiety and lower inhibitions, but after that, drinking can make matters worse. The spirit may be more willing, but the body becomes less able: Alcohol is a nervous-system depressant and interferes with spinal reflexes necessary for sexual response.

Using other recreational drugs to siphon off stress may also have drawbacks. Marijuana, like alcohol, can lower inhibitions, but it also dries mucous membranes. And tranquilizers reduce sympathetic-nervous-system activity and may therefore interfere with orgasm and ejaculation.

TRANSITION TIME

Then what should you do if stress is damping your sex life? Sometimes nothing. Loss of sexual desire is a natural response to a crisis or a temporary pressure, says San Francisco sex therapist and author Lonnie Barbach. A new baby in the family may put sex on hold for a while. A move or the loss of a job may also dampen ardor.

Our bodies are programmed to react to a crisis by shutting down nonessential functions and conserving energy. "We're not intended to carry on reproductive functions when we're in danger or threatened," explains New York's Dr. Helen Singer Kaplan, an authority on sexual disorders.

Once the stressful situation ends, sexual interest is likely to return. But in the meantime, it is important not to attribute what is essentially a time-management problem (say, job overload) to a personal failing in the other person ("He's self-centered"; "She's cold") that's never bothered you before. Blame—rejection—and before you know it, the relationship is poisoned.

Another kind of stress is ongoing—built into a job or domestic situation. Many people actually create chronic stress by their personal and professional choices, says Dr. Barbach. If your life is making you irritable or tired, she says, overhaul it or reconcile yourself to an impoverished sex life.

Other therapists feel the negative effects of stress can be minimized even when its source can't be eliminated. After a long, hard day, people are often full of "negative energy," which is subjectively quite different from the positive energy of anticipation, says psychologist-author Bernie Zilbergeld of Oakland, California. If they immediately launch into domestic duties and chores, they ricochet from one type of stress to another. He recommends a transition period: Set aside a regular time to settle into being together. Chat, stroll, have a glass of wine (but not more). Says Dr. Zilbergeld, "A few minutes of peace and quiet can be worth four hours of foreplay."

Some people also need a *personal* transition before they can enjoy being with someone else. It can be spent exercising, reading the paper, listening to music, working at a hobby, bathing, meditating—any activity that says good-bye to the workday.

PLAYFUL PLEASURES

The first step in "turning on" is to turn off the day's pressures and achieve that relaxed yet heightened state that sets the stage for intimacy. The specific strategies that follow here are designed to restore a sense of play to your life and help you relax. These techniques, of course, are not meant to replace professional counseling for serious relationship problems or sexual inhibition.

Review Priorities

How important is sex in your life? People may feel pressured to give it too much time and attention, especially if they are trying to live up to some standard of frequency. Then sex itself becomes a source of stress, one more duty to cross off the "to do" list. The solution may be to decide it's fine for sex to take a backseat.

But if sex does have high priority, you can learn to put aside less highly valued activities when Eros calls. This is easier said than done, especially when couples cannot agree on the priorities. As San Francisco psychiatrist Harvey Caplan observes, stress is best seen as a shared problem: "Both partners need to be on the same side of the issue. If they can't eliminate stress from their lives, they can at least cooperate to work around it."

Make Dates
Single people must set aside time for their "social life." Married couples and those living together can often benefit by doing the same—by scheduling "dates" with each other. Knowing that certain hours are reserved solely for fun and games, sexual or otherwise, can help unhook you from other obligations. The date can be made days ahead, but psychologist Carol Rinkleib Ellison of Oakland, California, also recommends issuing an invitation in the morning for an evening tête-à-tête: "If you light the pilot early," she says, "the furnace can warm up all day."

Some people worry that scheduling sex will stifle spontaneity. But Dr. Ellison notes that a date can be seen as time set aside for spontaneity. "As a sex therapist," she says, "I sometimes function as a sexual choreographer. I help people see that by deliberately taking care of details in advance—like buying the massage oil or sending the kids to the movies—they free themselves to be spontaneous later on."

Create a Context
There's nothing inherently wrong with the quickie, but if your life is a pressure cooker, it may pay to create a setting that puts you in a romantic or erotic mood—candlelight and music, erotic movies, sharing sexual fantasies, or wearing sexy underwear. Some people find it helps to make love somewhere besides the bedroom, or at times other than late evening.

Turn the Pressure Off
If you are under stress, the last thing you want to do is allow yourself or a partner to impose sexual-performance demands on you. When people feel they *must* have sex to please someone, they often have difficulty functioning at all. They detach themselves, becoming spectators instead of participants.

Sex therapists try to assure their clients that not every sexual interlude must include intercourse; nor need it involve orgasm. Efforts to "achieve" orgasm, no matter what your mood, can turn the joy of sex into the job of sex.

Following a strategy first proposed by Masters and Johnson, sex therapists often impose a temporary ban on intercourse and assign sensate-focus exercises for their clients. These exercises, which require a partner, are based on gentle, erotic massage. Typically, the couple agrees to avoid intercourse and orgasm during the period of days or weeks in which the assignments are carried out. The purpose of this ban is to remove performance pressure and to eliminate the fear of failure. Many couples have never spent a protracted period of time simply playing sensually with a lover. Stroking and caressing, if they have occurred at all, have been regarded as a means to an end—orgasm or ejaculation—rather than valuable activities in their own right.

Sensate-focus exercises can be adapted by couples who do not have specific sexual problems but find that stress has carried over into the bedroom, sabotaging the experience. Incorporating the leisurely exchange of pleasure into lovemaking can help you relax and establish an erotic mood. If afterward you discuss what you liked and disliked, you and your partner may learn something new about erotic preferences. And an occasional agreement to forgo intercourse and perhaps orgasm, or to make these experiences optional, will allow you to revel in the kind of low-keyed playfulness many hard-driving, goal-oriented people deny themselves. Sex then becomes a refuge from stress instead of yet another source of it. On p. 139, you'll find some simple guidelines to help you get started.

"Reframe" the Experience
Another strategy may be to view sex in a different light—to reframe it mentally. Busy people sometimes feel, consciously or not, that despite its pleasures, sex is an intrusion that uses up valuable time and energy. But it may be useful to regard sex as a way of recharging your batteries. As one man once put it, after orgasm he

Sensate Focus: Relaxing for Love

There is no magic list of procedures to follow for sensate-focus exercises, but there are some general guidelines. It's pleasant to shower or bathe first; use massage oil or skin lotion if you wish. Eliminate potential distractions—take the phone off the hook. You may decide to set time limits or simply continue as long as both partners wish. As part of sex therapy, sensate-focus sessions typically occur in two phases: In the first sessions there is no touching of the genital area or the woman's breasts; in the second phase, touching of these areas is allowed. You may or may not want to experiment with this sequence.

At the start of each session one partner should volunteer to act first as the giver of pleasure. Sometimes, "who goes first" as giver or receiver is an issue to be negotiated. Some people cannot feel relaxed about receiving pleasure until they have "paid their dues" by first giving pleasure. Others feel annoyed at having to "provide service" unless they have first received.

If you are the receiver, start by stretching out on your stomach; later, turn over on your back. Feel free to be completely "selfish," and don't worry about whether the giver is getting bored or tired. How you handle communication is up to both of you. The receiver may agree to accept whatever the giver offers without comment, unless the giver does something annoying or unpleasant. That way the giver, too, can become fully involved in his or her own experience. Or you may decide that the receiver will provide a running commentary on what feels good and offer gentle, tactful suggestions when the giver does something unpleasant, irritating, or simply ineffective.

If you are the giver, one way to start is to slowly massage or caress the head, neck, and shoulders, then gradually work down to the back, arms, and hands, buttocks, legs, and feet. But modify this strategy as you wish. Be creative. You can use your lips and hair as well as your hands if that feels comfortable.

While caressing, the giver should, to use Masters and Johnson's term, "give to get": The giver not only provides a pleasant experience for the other partner but also learns which kinds of stroking and touching he or she finds most pleasurable. The giver also notices his or her personal response to the smell, texture, and temperature of various parts of the lover's body. You may discover that sensual touching without trying to achieve orgasm opens a whole new world of erotic experience.

When a session is to include genital touching, begin with nongenital touching and then go on to gentle stroking of the genitals and the woman's breasts. Take your time. Since there's no goal in sensate focus except relaxed pleasure, you can stay with an activity as long as you both enjoy it.

During genital stimulation, you might want to try positions originally recommended by Masters and Johnson. When the woman is stimulating the man, he lies on his back and puts his legs over hers as she sits facing him. When the man is stimulating the woman, he sits with his back against the headboard, and she sits with her back against him, so that both are facing the same way. In these positions, the receiver can easily signal a desire for a change in pressure, direction, position, or rate of stroking by gently guiding the giver's hand with the receiver's own. But verbal instructions are fine, too.

Whether or not you decide to go on to intercourse, sensate focus will be most effective in reducing stress if neither partner pressures the other to be responsive. The giver should simply provide sensual pleasure and emotional support, all the while enjoying the experience of giving. If anxiety, embarrassment, or other negative responses occur, they can be used as an opportunity for discussing and working through problems in the relationship. Serious negative reactions, however, may indicate a need for professional counseling.

For most people, giving and receiving sensory pleasure in a nondemanding context does more than simply increase awareness of sensation. Touch is one of the ways human beings show one another their innermost feelings, and touching that is tender and loving strengthens the emotional attachment between people. Therefore you may find that sensate-focus exercises add a special emotional dimension to physical intimacy.

Has Stress Zapped Your Sex Life?

Are stress and tension unwanted guests in your bedroom? Here's a checklist to help you and your partner take stock. Check those statements that are *usually* or *increasingly true* for each of you. If you make a copy and each of you checks it off separately, you can compare notes and use the responses as a springboard for heart-to-heart talks.

But remember, this is not a test; there is no "passing" or "failing" score. The statements merely highlight warning signals and are not intended to turn sex into another source of stress.

☐ Making love seems more trouble than it's worth.

☐ I'd like to have sex more often, but chores and responsibilities make that difficult.

☐ While making love I find myself thinking about work, family, or personal problems.

☐ I feel impatient when my partner takes a long time to become aroused or to have an orgasm.

☐ We make love when I am mentally or physically tired.

☐ I depend on alcohol or tranquilizers to relax me in advance.

☐ During sex I feel guilty about taking time out from other duties.

☐ My partner and I start without spending time together nonsexually.

☐ "Fooling around" without having intercourse seems pointless.

☐ When my partner takes the initiative, I feel he or she is making demands on my time or energy.

☐ Right after orgasm I feel an urge to jump up and get on with some other activity.

☐ My partner and I do not set any special time aside to be together.

☐ Sex is fine, but I get anxious if it goes into "overtime."

☐ Despite my interest, I have trouble switching from a nonerotic to an erotic mood.

☐ My partner and I make love late at night after everything else has been taken care of.

☐ Children, phone calls, or visitors keep interfering with our privacy.

☐ I am completely content with my sex life. *If both of you check this item, you can probably ignore your responses to all the others.*

feels his "molecules are realigned" and his head is clearer.

Zilbergeld and Ellison used reframing successfully in therapy with a work-driven man in his late twenties. Bob enjoyed sex but afterward regretted that he hadn't been doing work brought home from the office. Ambivalence caused him to resent his wife Mary's frequent sexual overtures, and eventually he refused to have sex. Though they cared greatly for each other, the relationship deteriorated.

Their therapy included many of the strategies described here. In addition, it was suggested to Bob that being with Mary could help him unwind and replenish his energy. He was asked to note the times during the day when he felt slightly excited or restless and to consider how doing something with Mary—touching, holding, loving—might help restore his concentration. In Mary's absence Bob was to let his feelings "simmer on the back burner," returning briefly to them so they would stay alive. Gradually, Bob learned to regard sex as an appropriate response to restlessness.

Reframing was also used with Mary, who tended to use sex for nonsexual purposes—to fight off bad moods, get attention, or bolster her ego. Eventually, she learned to use other methods to meet some of these needs. Mary became less compulsive about sex, Bob learned the value of play, and each came to enjoy the other more—both in and out of bed.

Rechannel Your Energy

Finally, when life's pressures get out of hand, it may help to schedule sex to take advantage of times when you are already aroused in a positive way. One couple that got a charge out of watching football on TV usually made love at halftime. The physical arousal generated by some activity can also be mentally associated with sex. Zilbergeld and Ellison tell of a woman who was a tennis ace: When she swung a tennis racket in her bedroom, the alternating tension and relaxation in her movements produced an exhilaration that spilled over into lovemaking. Tennis, anyone?

The strategies in this chapter are designed to rescue you from a headlong race through your daily schedule. School's out; it's time to play. But aside from the obvious value of a vibrant sex life, let's not forget that satisfying sex is itself one of the great mental and physical relaxers. It's one resource a relaxed body ought not forgo.

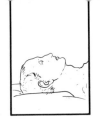

Chapter 13

A Good Night's Sleep

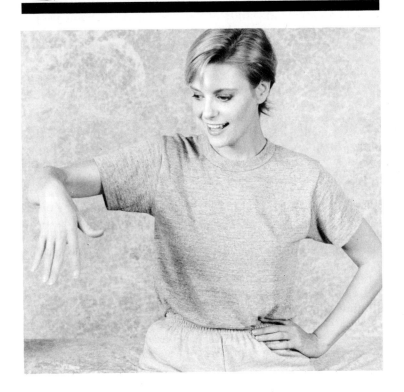

It's been a foggy, foul-tempered day. You nearly fell asleep in the office, on the way home from work, and watching TV after dinner. You look at the clock. At last, you can relax. You climb into bed for some desperately needed shut-eye. . . . Suddenly, you're wide awake. Once again, an endless night of tossing and turning is about to feed into a miserable, "underslept" day. How can you have a relaxed body? You've got insomnia!

According to a national survey, one of every three American adults reports having some difficulty falling asleep, staying asleep, or both. And because most of us have insomnia in times of stress, sleeplessness is usually held to be "in the mind."

But the conventional wisdom is wrong. Psychological stress and psychiatric ills such as depression account for only half of all cases of insomnia, according to a nationwide study of more than eight thousand persons with sleep disorders. At the same time, stress at some period in your life may establish a poor-sleep habit that goes on to have a life of its own.

"Insomnia is a symptom," explains Dr. Howard Roffwarg, director of the Sleep-Wake Disorders Center at Presbyterian Hospital in Dallas. "Like fever or stomachache, it requires a diagnosis." And that often involves a visit to a doctor savvy about sleep or to one of the nation's fast-growing sleep-disorders centers (see "Resources," p.189).

Physical ailments, such as sleep apnea (troubled breathing), repetitive leg jerks, a mix of waking and sleeping brain activity, and backup of stomach contents into the esophagus can produce restless nights. Sleeping pills may actually aggravate some of these disorders, particularly sleep apnea, potentially life-threatening interruptions in breathing.

Other culprits include caffeine, alcohol, and medications, as well as erratic hours—a fast-paced social life or frequent job-shift changes. A few "insomniacs" are simply five-or-six-hour sleepers, laboring under the misconception that they "need" eight hours.

But even after physical ills and other specific reasons for poor sleep are ruled out, insomnia can be a tough nut to crack. How long it's been going on is a key distinction in tailoring therapy. Experts now classify insomnia in three categories:

Transient insomnia may last a few days and is triggered by excitement, temporary jitters, or travel—Christmas Eve, the night before a key meeting or surgery, jet lag. Most people make up for the lost sleep in a few days.

Short-term insomnia—up to three weeks—is common in times of personal stress or serious medical illness. In some cases a doctor may prescribe sleeping pills for just a night or two to help weather the crisis.

Chronic insomnia, on the other hand, may persist for years. Some people are more prone to insomnia in times of stress, just as others may develop ulcers or headaches, says Dr. Peter Hauri, codirector of Dartmouth's sleep center. Yet many insomniacs carry no more than an average load of everyday anxieties but still become mired in poor sleep. Their problem is "learned insomnia."

Psychologist Hauri sketches a common scenario: Most of us sleep badly during a crisis. For some, a few wretched nights—and exhausted days—turn not sleeping into a special worry. The more they try, the more sleep eludes them. Cues in and around the bedroom—darkness, pillows, brushing their teeth—gradually are associated with frustration and arousal. Now the sleep stakes start to escalate.

Such people often drift off when they don't want to—watching TV or driving, for example. They may also fall asleep on the living-room couch, away from home, or, unlike most people, in the slightly uncomfortable confines of a sleep lab.

For some people a predisposition to suffer

an occasional poor night's sleep may be all it takes to fuel lifelong insomnia. You can't learn not to worry about sleep if a few "naturally occurring" bad nights a month reinforce this anxiety, says Hauri.

No pill yet invented will cure chronic insomnia, says Hauri. In recent years U.S. physicians have been writing fewer sleeping-pill prescriptions and are more sophisticated about when and what they do prescribe. In 1971 doctors churned out 42 million prescriptions; by 1982, the most recent count, this figure was halved.

But if sleep is your sorrow, you don't have to rely on a pill and deal with its next-day side effects to make peace with Morpheus. Sleep researchers now offer an extensive smorgasbord of do-it-yourself techniques to induce slumber. By the time you drop off to sleep, one way or another, mind and body must finally relax their grip on the day.

Direct relaxation techniques are not the only way to unwind for sleep. If your hours are erratic, you may wish to check out your "sleep hygiene" and give your biological clocks a break. If your mind races once the lights go out, investigate "cognitive focusing" or other distraction techniques. If physical tension is the problem, relaxation methods may be right for you.

One caveat: Not all insomniacs are psychologically or physiologically tense, Dr. Hauri points out. "People who are relaxed in both spheres but still unable to sleep may actually become worse when pushed into relaxation training," he says. (See "When Relaxing Is Unrelaxing," p.18.) It's important to rule out physical causes of insomnia and make certain that relaxation training is your cup of tea.

You may have to hopscotch between techniques to find what works for you. But be patient as you experiment. It's rather like dieting, explains Stanford psychologist Richard Coleman. People who do well on a diet are usually those who follow a structured program. Similarly, a few days of a sleep regimen is seldom effective. It takes about five weeks to see improvement, he says. And all the experts emphasize that no single technique works for everyone, nor does any single method top the list.

If tension and stress are keeping you awake or if poor sleep habits, conditioned by stress, make bed a battlefield, it may be time to clean up your sleep act. Here's a roundup of strategies sleep experts often prescribe:

SLEEP HYGIENE

Some people, says Hauri, can break all the sleep-hygiene rules, yet fall asleep anytime, anyplace; others must take care to heed sensible guidelines.

Do:

■ Get up at about the same time seven days a week. This helps keep internal biological clocks synchronized. Going to bed at the same time is less critical; you can't force yourself to sleep if you're not sleepy.

■ Get enough sleep to feel refreshed, but don't try to squeeze the last drop of sleep out of every night.

■ Keep a daily sleep log. Just as recording every mouthful helps dieters, documenting sleep habits often shows where your weak spots are.

■ Set up presleep rituals. In the same way bedtime stories help kids settle down, simple routines can help psych you into sleep. But to break an insomniac habit, start fresh with new routines. Check the doors, set out tomorrow's clothes, assume a specific sleep posture, indulge in a pleasant fantasy.

■ Exercise regularly, preferably in the late afternoon; avoid vigorous exercise after 6 P.M. (Sex at bedtime doesn't count as "vigorous" exercise. What's more, most people find orgasm a terrific sleep inducer.)

■ Soundproof and light-proof your bedroom. You never get used to traffic or airplane din; the noise disturbs sleep, even if you don't awaken completely. If necessary, mask sounds with "white" noise from an air conditioner or electric fan.

■ Adjust room temperature to suit yourself; the comfort range is huge and no single setting is best for everyone.

■ Eat with sleep in mind. A high-carbohydrate supper, such as pasta, may foster sleepiness; a light bedtime snack may keep hunger pangs from awakening you during the night. Warm milk at bedtime has good folklore credentials.

■ Keep busy, even after a sleepless night. The greater your sleep deficit, the more you need large-body activity, like walking or house-cleaning, instead of fine-muscle activity, such as needlepoint or complex mental tasks.

Don't:

■ Consume caffeine after 4 P.M. or smoke at bedtime—nicotine is a stimulant, too.
■ Take a nip at bedtime. Alcohol may relax and ease you into sleep, but it may also cause frequent awakenings in the latter half of the night.
■ Nap—unless you know that naps leave you refreshed and won't interfere with sleep.

SLEEP RESTRICTION

Insomniacs often spend too much time in bed, says psychologist Arthur Spielman, director of the Sleep Disorders Center at the City College of New York. In a misguided effort to make up for lost sleep, they may start going to bed earlier and earlier, logging eight, nine, or more hours in bed. But they're miserable because they sleep only five or six hours.

To decondition patients for whom bed is as good as an alarm clock, Spielman and a team at New York's Montefiore Hospital tried reverse psychology. They limited time in bed to only the hours patients actually sleep. Thirty-five chronic insomniacs tracked their sleep habits for two weeks. Then the average amount of sleep patients got was "prescribed" as the maximum amount of time they were permitted to stay in bed.

Every morning for the next six weeks, participants phoned the researchers to report how much sleep they got. Those who slept at least 90 percent of their time in bed during a five-day period were rewarded with an extra fifteen minutes' bedtime each night. However, "non-efficient" sleepers were penalized by having

time in bed reduced. By the study's end nearly all the insomniacs were sleeping better and longer.

Do-it-yourself sleep restriction takes lots of motivation, Spielman says. You may have to cut two or more hours from the time you spend in bed. His advice: Stay up later at night, but get up at the same time each morning, including weekends; no napping or resting during the day. After you begin to sleep better—typically within a week or two—boost time in bed by not more than fifteen minutes. As soon as you are awake less than thirty minutes for five consecutive nights, give yourself another fifteen minutes.

STIMULUS CONTROL

The aim in this technique, somewhat related to sleep restriction, is to neutralize bedroom antisleep stimuli. Dr. Richard Bootzin, chairman of psychology at Northwestern University, suggests:
■ Go to bed only when you are sleepy. If your spouse or partner is ready for sleep and you're not, go into the other room to read or watch TV. No lights-out law says two people must retire at the same time.
■ Reserve your bed and bedroom for sleep and sex only. No reading, TV, or curling up to talk on the phone. Don't pay bills or work in the bedroom either. And try to keep arguments with your partner out of the bedroom.
■ If you're not asleep in ten or fifteen minutes, go into another room. Do some quiet activity—reading or watching TV. Though a single high-carbohydrate snack may induce drowsiness, do not keep snacking lest eating become a reward for sleeplessness.
■ Go back to bed only when you are sleepy; get up again and leave your bedroom if you can't sleep.
■ Set an alarm clock and get up at the same time every day no matter how you slept. Don't "sleep in" on weekends—at least not more than an hour or two.
■ Don't nap during the day. Even if you're tired, tough it out till bedtime.

COGNITIVE FOCUSING

Psychologist Patricia Lacks of Washington University in St. Louis says the injunction to get out of bed whenever you're not sleeping is more than some people can handle. But substituting mental diversions to banish unwanted thoughts may help.

Telling yourself "Don't think about it" may be futile unless you intentionally think about something else, Lacks explains. Fortunately, you can't focus on two things simultaneously. The trick is to shift your focus. "Imagine you are a TV set," she suggests. "You can block out channel 9 by tuning in channel 11."

Choose a focus technique that appeals to you. Then briefly practice using it for focus control during the day so you can turn it on readily during the night. Here are some simple suggestions:

■ Focus on your physical surroundings or on an interesting task. Count floor or ceiling tiles, examine the construction of a piece of furniture, read, watch TV.

■ Focus on a train of thought that fully diverts your mind. Recite a poem, do mental arithmetic such as multiplication tables or counting backward from one thousand by threes; count sheep (it works); list categories of animals, birds, or countries alphabetically; compose a long "letter" to someone; invent a fantasy.

■ Focus on body sensations. Where do you feel cold, pressure, tingling? Various relaxation techniques used for insomnia may owe their success to their ability to harness a wandering mind as well as to the physical relaxation they induce.

■ Try imagery. Conjure up a beach scene. Recall the pleasant warmth of the sun and the tranquilizing sound of the waves. Go for a mental stroll down a familiar path. "Try to be inside your scene rather than outside watching yourself," Lacks advises.

MONOTONOUS STIMULATION

Most people find the sound of ocean waves, raindrops, a fan, or a heartbeat soothing, even soporific. In a sleep-lab study, listening to alternating on-off tones helped people fall asleep faster than either total silence or a monotonous sound. Tones worked even better when people counted them, a task demanding enough to drive out unwanted thoughts. Yes, just like counting sheep.

RELAXATION

Spending time with any of your favorite relaxation techniques may be a direct way to tackle insomnia. The many relaxation routines in this book offer an extra advantage: They require you to schedule time for destressing your daily life. Thus, beyond their specific relaxation benefit, these techniques automatically distract your mind from petty, niggling worries and transport you to wider, more soothing horizons.

■ Regular exercise—swimming, running, weight lifting, walking, aerobic dancing, tennis—is a natural relaxer. But avoid evening sessions.

■ You may find the muscle-feedback techniques—progressive relaxation (see p.12) and the body scan (see p.13)—perfect preludes to a good night's sleep. Perhaps meditation (see p.17) is more your style or autogenic suggestion (see p.16). Experiment and see whether they're right for you.

Sleep Stretches

And now a perfect bedtime treat. It's hard to fall asleep if your body hurts. As part of your winding-down routine you may wish to devote a quiet period to a pleasant mixture of gentle movements. Here's a practical routine, developed by Lilias Folan of Cincinnati, who teaches yoga and relaxation to millions over public television. Not only do these sleep stretches ease aches and tension, but they also provide a fresh prebedtime routine, free of antisleep conditioning.

Start with your *upper body*. Stand tall, relax your shoulders, and plant your feet on the ground. Let your arms hang heavy. Feel as if someone has painlessly lifted you up by a few hairs at the top of your head. Rest one hand on the back of a chair for balance. After each exercise, pause to enjoy the relaxed sensation.

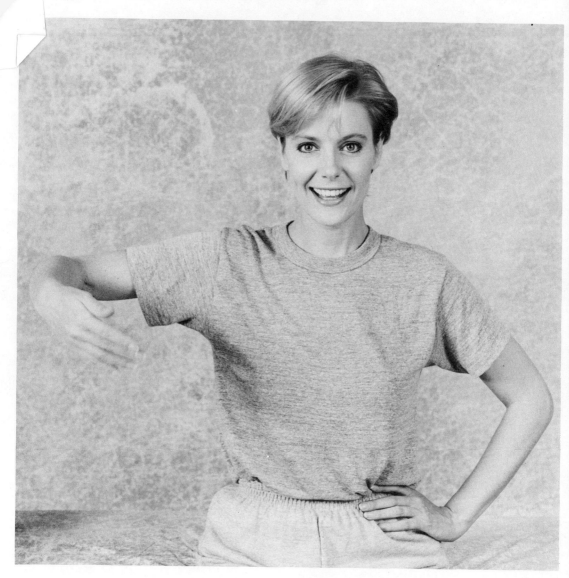

Arm Shake
Soften your knees as you bend forward to release your lower back. Shake your right arm.
Slowly at first, then more vigorously. Shake
your hand and fingers, the elbow, the whole
arm. Repeat on the opposite side.

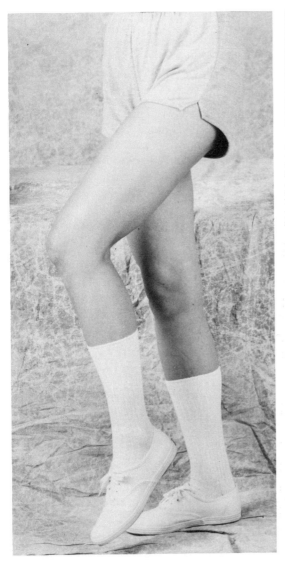

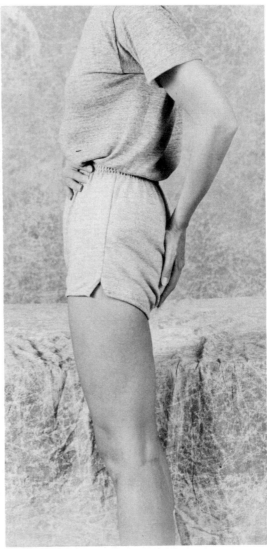

Leg Shake
Shake your foot first and work up to the thigh. Slowly, then more vigorously.

Pelvis Tilt
Exhale, and contract your pelvic muscles. Now inhale, release, and relax.

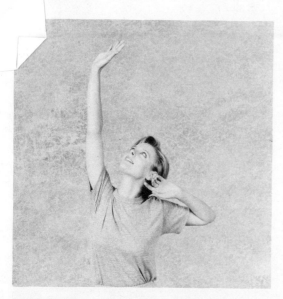

Star Reach
Raise your arms above your head and reach!
Not too high at first. Then higher.

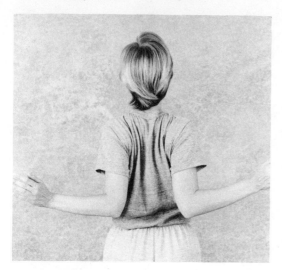

Lemon Squeeze
Inhale, then exhale and try to touch elbows
behind your back. You won't be able to, but
imagine you are squeezing a lemon between
both shoulder blades. Hold. Don't strain. Release, relax, and enjoy the feeling.

Chest Expander
Clasp your hands behind you. Straighten your
elbows and pull your shoulders down from
your ears. Slowly raise your arms. Open your
chest; lift the breastbone and chin; squeeze an
imaginary lemon. Now inhale, and tighten the
buttock muscles. Pause, exhale, release slowly,
and relax your arms. Observe the lightness in
your arms and shoulders.

Next, some *back*- and *abdomen*-soothers.
Sit down with your knees well apart and your
feet on the ground.

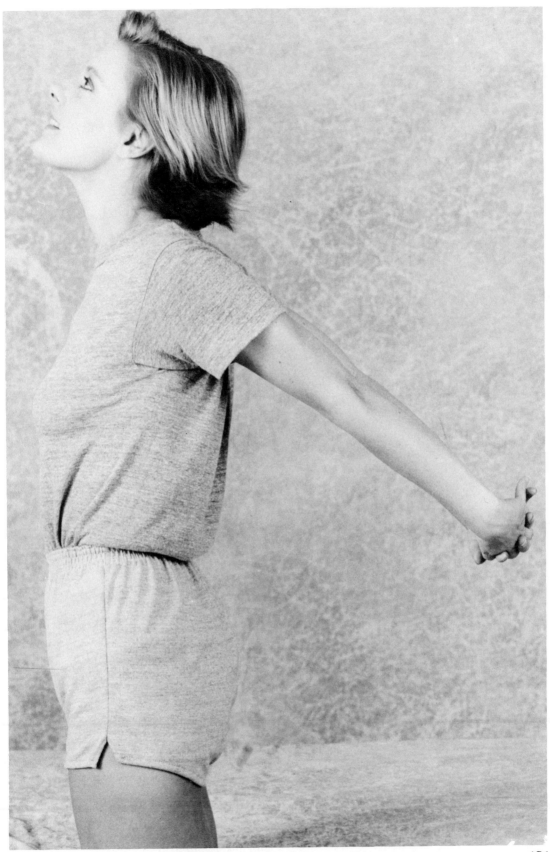

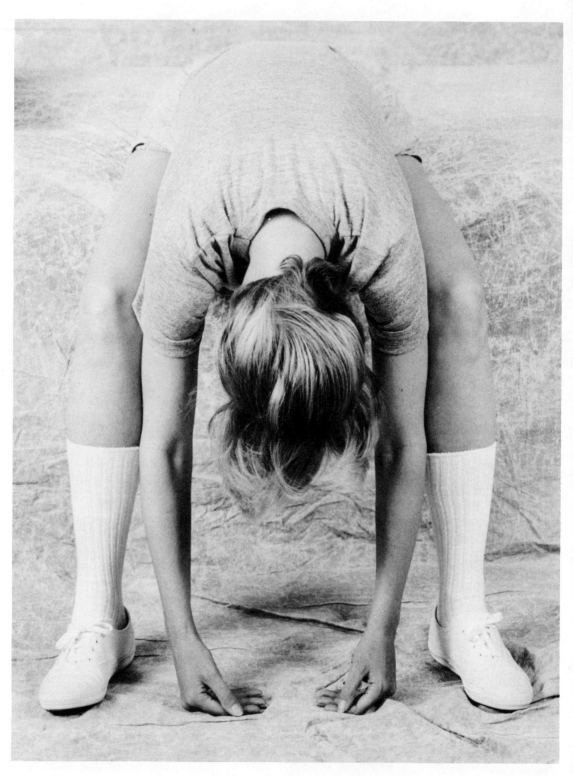

Forward Bend and Backward Arch
Raise your arms to the ceiling. Exhale, and
stretch forward from the hips. Bring the arms
down between the knees. Breathe comfortably.
Now inhale and arch back. Stretch! Exhale,
and lower your arms. Repeat.

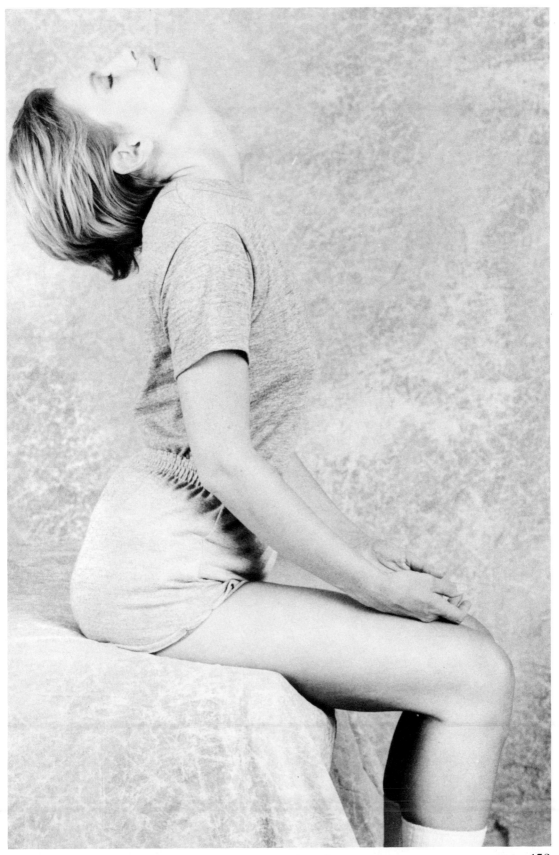

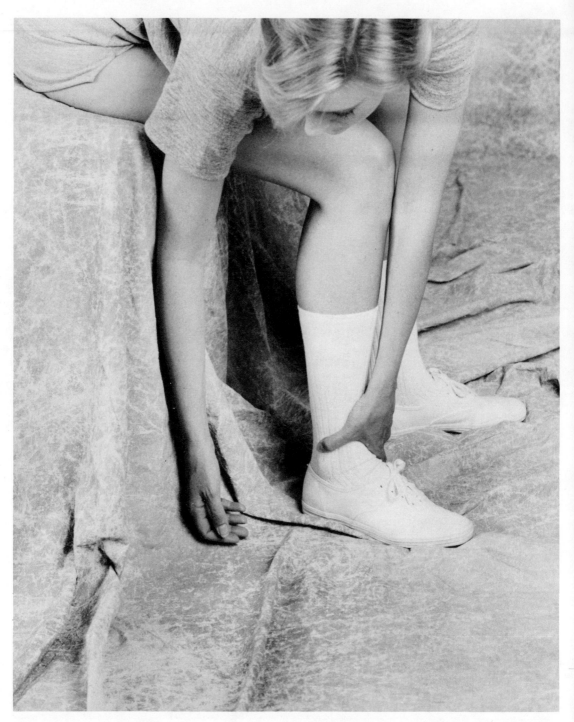

Seated Twist
Clasp your right ankle with the left hand. The right hand hangs limp. Inhale. Raise the right hand. Exhale. Bring it down. Let your eyes follow your fingertips. Reverse.

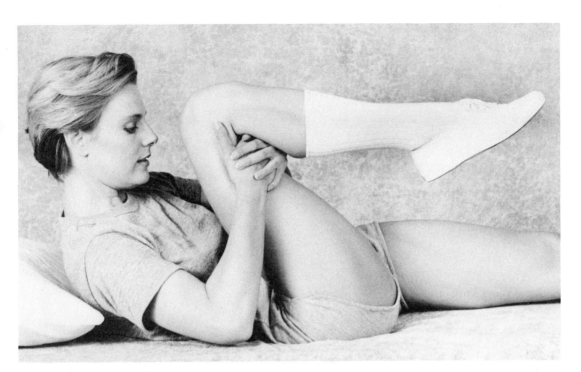

Knee to Chest

Lie down. Bend your right knee to your chest. Hands hold the leg behind the back of your thigh. Press the thigh to the chest a few times. Press again firmly, inhale; exhale slowly. Raise your head toward your knee. Pause, inhale, and release slowly. Exhale, head up, pause, and inhale, head down. Release the leg and repeat on the other side.

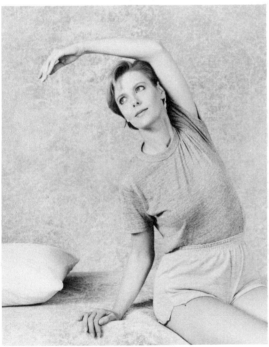

Side to Side

Raise your right arm so the upper arm is close to the ear. Relax the elbow. Inhale. Then exhale and bend left. Squeeze at the waist. Pause. Inhale and straighten up. Don't slump forward. Pause, exhale, and repeat. Repeat on the left side.

155

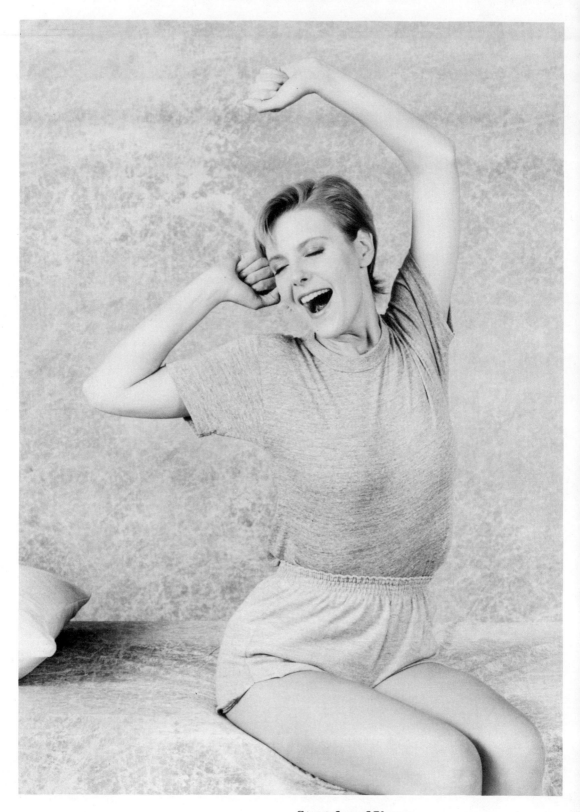

Stretch and Yawn
Open your mouth wide. Stretch the arms upward as you yawn. Repeat.

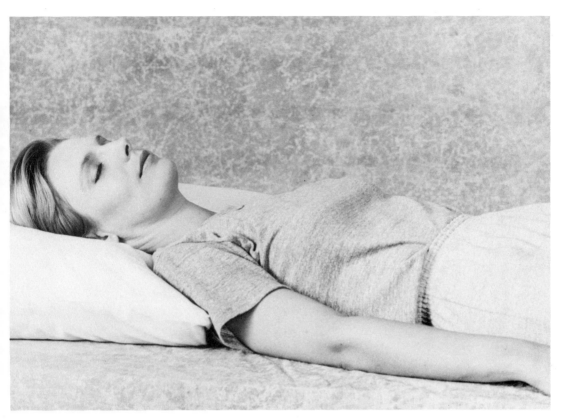

Relaxed Position

Imagine lying in a soft velvet hammock. Let the rhythm of your breath gently move it to and fro. It's a quiet spring evening. Hear the comforting sounds of night. Focus on your back. Let it sink heavily into the hammock. Sense that the small of your back and your neck are supported by softness.

Over and Out

Focus on your hands, your face, your jaw, around your legs, your knees, the soles of your feet. Let them soften; feel them relax. Give in to that comfortable, heavy, warm feeling. Let the soft, warm darkness flow around you. Time is suspended . . . quiet . . . sink deeper and deeper into the hammock.

The routes to a good night's sleep are many and varied, and not all involve relaxation itself. But healing sleep is essential to the nurture of a relaxed body. Sleep engenders energy, clarity, and optimism and provides the physical and emotional fuel needed to cope well with the day's demands. What did you say? . . . Yawn. . . . Your whole body feels soft, relaxed, warm, drowsy. . . . Your mind is calm, drifting. . . . Pleasant dreams . . . zzzzzz.

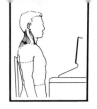

Chapter 14

Pain in the Office

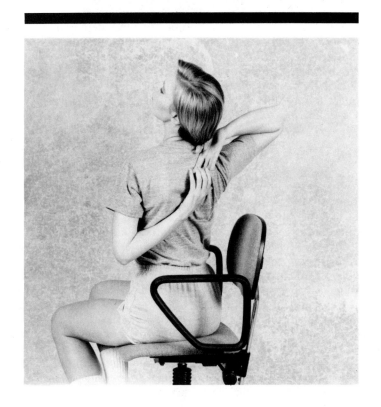

Not all the tension in the office can be blamed on the boss; office furniture and design are also culprits. Neck, shoulder, and back exercises can help relax abused muscles, and in the next chapter we will examine movement habits that produce stress and strain. But it also makes sense to inspect your workplace and tackle the problem at its source.

We are rapidly becoming a nation of sitters. By 1990, it's estimated, at least half of all U.S. office workers will use a word processor, a data processor, or some variant. There already are office systems designed to put information at your fingertips and intercoms so efficient that leaving your desk to communicate with a fellow office worker is impractical. But workers whose fingers do the walking via a computer terminal may pay a price when they try to stand up at the end of the day.

The sweeping changes in this white-collar—actually, "pink-collar"—revolution have caught management and its many stiff and sore employees off guard. "The typical American worker is no longer a man in a hard hat. She is a woman at a typewriter, or rather, a woman at a terminal," says Karen Nussbaum, director of "9 to 5," a national organization of working women.

Though office workers may not get clonked on the head by a steel girder, they have their own occupational injuries. Most of these reflect too-intimate contact with their high-tech labor savers: eyestrain from glaring video screens, headaches from neck or shoulder tension, low-back problems from improperly adjusted chairs, and hand or arm pain from repeated contact with unpadded surfaces. Sitting for long periods is hard enough on the human body, but when unadjustable, procrustean office furniture forces the body to make all the adjustments, chronic injury may result.

These injuries are usually not as serious as industrial traumas, but the results are not too different: unhappiness on the job, time away from work, and insurance claims for problems that won't go away. A workplace that has not evolved as fast as its technology may end up creating a chamber of environmental stress.

The science of making the hole fit the peg is dubbed "ergonomics" (ergo = work). Its real start in this country came with World War II and the need for well-designed fighter-plane cockpits. Gradually, human engineering moved into other military areas such as tank design and, understandably, into the space program.

Only in the last decade, with its sweeping changes in office technology, has ergonomics been invited into the office and other areas of civilian life—kitchen and bathroom, for example. Computers have wrought the most important change in office life since typewriters, telephones, and mimeograph machines transformed the earlier Charles Dickensian office, says Allen Weston, Columbia University professor of law and government.

To stem the problems of the new technology, many companies have started their own "human-factors" departments. Others have hired outside firms to come in and redesign tools or the entire work space. Though some firms—IBM, Kodak, AT&T, to name a few—have established human-factors departments to deal with problems *before* they develop, the ergonomics troops are usually summoned to rescue environments already seriously in trouble. There may be an eyestrain epidemic or a major outbreak of backaches or other muscular-skeletal problems. The desperate management will then call in the human-factors people.

"Unfortunately, if it's not broken, people don't think they have to fix it," says Carole Hunter, founder of Industrial Biomechanics, an ergonomic consulting firm in North Carolina. "There is nothing more difficult than trying to convince a company executive they need you. They usually have to find out for themselves." The human-factors folks are quick to point out that a data-processing system intended to streamline a company's operations won't be efficient unless workers are comfortable. Once the ergonomics experts move in, the before-after contrast can be striking. Here are some examples:

■ At a data-management facility in the South, employees responsible for filing the magnetic tapes had an unusual number of shoulder and back injuries. Since the tapes weighed a mere two and a half pounds each and the employees were all in their twenties and early thirties, it didn't make sense.

Hunter came in and found that most of the tape librarians carried as many as fourteen tapes with one hand while they filed them with the other. These workers handled up to eight hundred tapes a day in this fashion.

Solution: Hunter designed a tape cart that

held more tapes than a librarian could manage, increased the efficiency of the operation, and eliminated shoulder injuries. The cost: $200 a cart.

■ A VDT operator in the tape library of Aetna Life Insurance was plagued with eyestrain. Karen Assunto of the company's people/technology department was asked to do some sleuthing. She discovered that glare from the overhead lights was dimming the screen, causing the operator to compensate by turning the terminal's light up.

Solution: Assunto removed two banks of lights above the operator's desk. No more eye problem. The cost: nothing.

"These are all cheap and easy fixes," says Assunto. "And in many cases the simple fixes are the most successful." Indeed, for economic reasons they may also be the best way to start.

Aetna, for instance, is replacing difficult-to-adjust chairs with ergonomic chairs with easy-to-reach controls. The company is also considering an easily adjustable table for workers in the claims department. "But we're bringing them in slowly because the cost of installing four thousand new tables and chairs would be prohibitive," says Assunto. "In the meantime, we're showing people how to use existing materials to adjust their environment. They appreciate knowing they have some control over their work conditions."

To help you take the hurt out of your work space, ergonomics expert Hunter describes what to look for in well-behaved office furniture and offers some tips on how to avoid terminal agony. Cosmetically, homegrown fixes may not stand up to the high-tech dazzle of the new ergonomic "work stations" now available, but they embody the same principles—and cost pennies by contrast.

THE CHAIR

The key to adapting the hole to the peg is adjustability. In this sense the real ergonomic "hot seat" is literally the office chair. By changing its dimensions to fit your needs, you can alleviate much of the stress and strain that goes hand-in-hand with a tough day at the office.

New "ergonomic" office chairs are equipped with easy hand controls so you can adjust your chair with a flick of the wrist. But if you're stuck with an old-model chair, don't be lazy—you can make some improvements. Get down on your hands and knees and turn the under-seat screw that adjusts height. You may

also be able to change the backrest angle.

An ergonomically sound chair should be able to go as low as fifteen inches and as high as twenty-one inches to fit people of different height. Your elbows should bend at about ninety degrees or slightly more, says Hunter. "If your elbow is at less than ninety degrees, you'll have to hike your shoulders up, which will cause tension."

Tension accumulates in the lower back, too. Leaning against the chair's backrest as often as possible is one way to give your back the support it needs. To use the backrest properly, adjust it so it reclines no more than twenty degrees. On the other hand, less than twenty degrees probably defeats its purpose, which is to let you lean back and take some of the pressure off your spine. The backrest should be adjusted to any height that feels good. "Studies show that placing the support anywhere along the curve of the lower back is fine," says Hunter. If your chair won't accommodate to your back, tie a small pillow or piece of foam to the chair back to provide low-back support.

Then there's the "settling slope" of the seat. If you are buying a chair, look for a slight backward slant, about five degrees; it will keep you from slipping forward. Ideally, your hips should be at a ninety-degree angle and so should your knees. But the slant should not be too pronounced, because it may put pressure on the popliteal space—the area right behind the bend of the knee—and cut off circulation.

If your feet don't reach the floor, Hunter recommends using a footrest to bring your knees up to the ninety-degree angle. A large box weighted with old magazines will do in a pinch.

Also, spare those elbows. Chair arms should be well-padded to prevent elbow trauma. Do-it-yourselfers can wrap some foam around unfriendly chair arms.

ACCESS TO WORK STATION

The chair should be low enough and its arms designed so you have easy access to a desk or keyboard. Leaning forward all day to reach your work can cause a nasty backache.

Also, the edge of your desk or work surface should be rounded or padded. A sharp edge may cut into your arms or wrists and cause pressure on nerves.

VIEWING ANGLE

If you use a typewriter or a word processor with a fixed screen, you don't have much choice of viewing angle. But if the keyboard is separate from the screen, raise the screen so you can gaze more or less directly at it without bending your neck downward. Your eyes should not have to rotate more than twenty degrees in going from the screen to your work materials. These should be on about the same level as the screen. Keeping your neck in as neutral a position as possible, says Hunter, will avoid neck strain and eyestrain.

Ready-made stands that raise the screen to eye level are available at computer and office-supply stores, but it's easy to improvise. Prop the terminal screen up on a large solid box and place a copy stand atop another object—a double-tiered in-box will do.

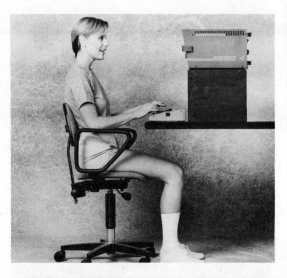

SCREEN GLARE

A major source of eyestrain is screen glare from sunlight or bright fluorescent lights that compete with the light from the screen.

To solve a possible sunlight problem, Hunter recommends installing window blinds on the offending windows. For glare from overhead lights, she suggests replacing the bright lights with weaker ones or extinguishing enough lights to reduce the screen washout.

Also available are screen hoods that fit over the screen like the visor of a baseball cap and shield it from other light sources.

DESKERCISES

Taming your office furniture isn't the whole story. The human body that spends its work-day tethered to a terminal or frozen in one position for long periods needs freedom and some thawing out. Ergonomics experts recommend frequent exercise breaks—thirty seconds to five minutes—throughout the day to prevent tension buildup.

According to one poll of 1,263 office workers, 36 percent worry about back pain. If your office is taking the sing and spring out of your body, you will find a wealth of healing moves in Chapters 7 through 9 of this book ("Neck-savers," "Backsavers," and "Backsoothers").

In addition, here's a special section of simple exercises you can do right at your desk. Designed to release nervous tension and increase blood flow and joint mobility, these exercises take about five to ten minutes. Before you start: If your chair has wheels and is inclined to slide, be sure the wheels are locked or wedged in place.

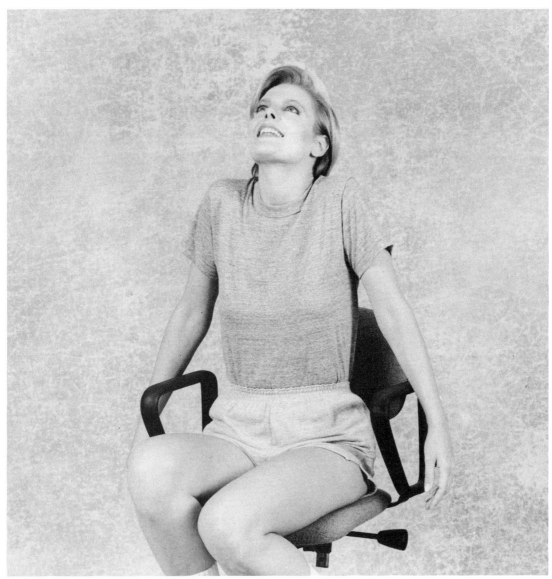

Shoulder Shrugs
Roll your shoulders five times in a circle, using
their full range of motion. Reverse direction.

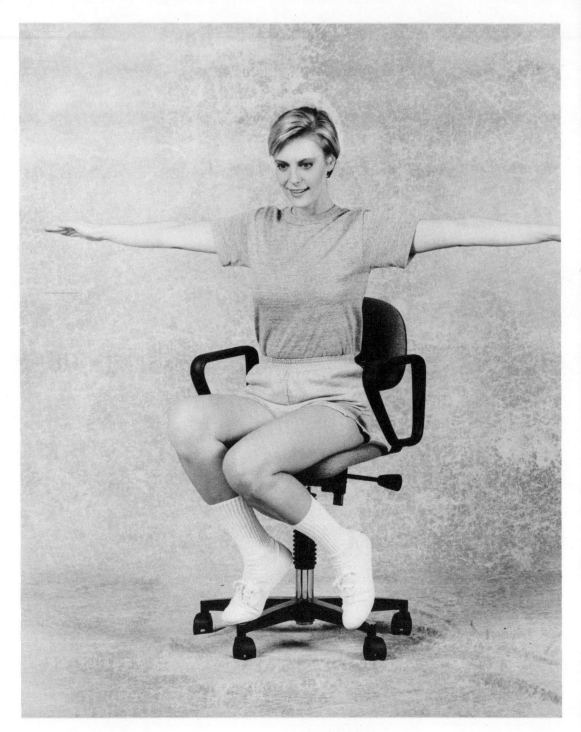

Arm Circles
Straighten your arms and raise them out to the side. Rotate your arms in small circles, forward and then backward.

Chest Stretch
Grasp your arms behind your neck and press your elbows backward until you feel your chest muscles pull. Relax and repeat.

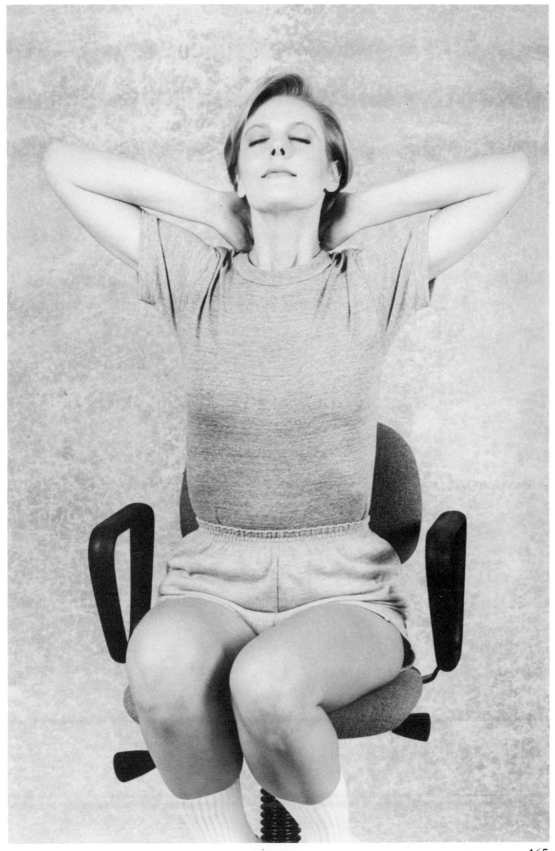

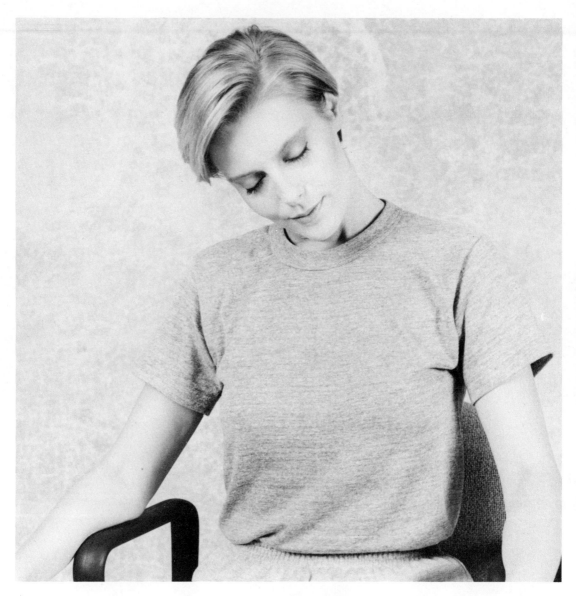

Neck Roll
Slowly let your head drop to the left and then to the right. Now drop it slowly to your chest; then raise your chin as high as you can. Turn your head all the way to the left; repeat to the right.

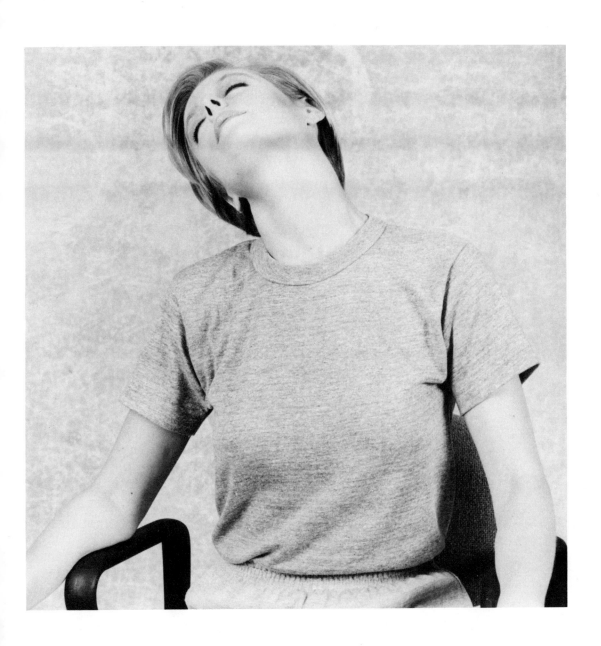

Upper-Back Stretch

With your hands on your shoulders, twist at the waist until you feel the stretch across your upper back. Return to center and twist the other way.

Side Stretch

Lock your fingers and lift your arms over your head until your elbows are straight. Slowly lean to the left, then the right. Feel the stretch in your sides.

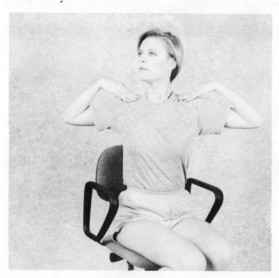

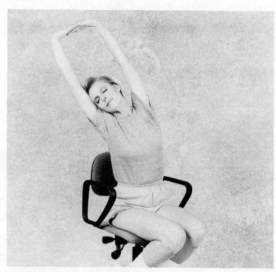

Shoulder Stretch

Reach over your upper back from above with your right hand and from below with your left hand. Try to hook the fingers of your two hands. Repeat on the other side.

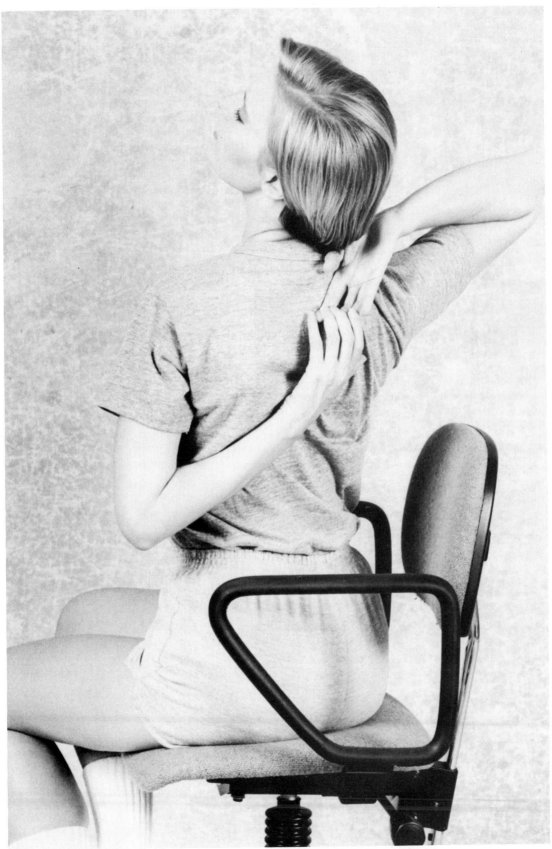

Wrist Twist

Extend one arm directly in front of your body. Use your other hand to bend the outstretched fingers upward until the wrist bends backward. Repeat with the opposite hand.

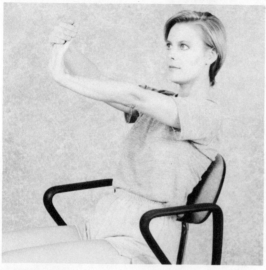

Finger Flex

Palms down, spread your thumbs and fingers as far apart as you can. Hold for the count of five and relax.

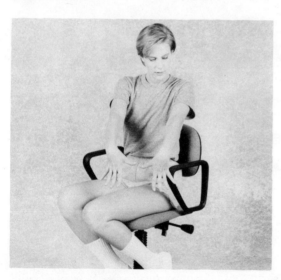

Hug

Cross your arms in front of your chest and touch your shoulder blades. Hug yourself—you deserve it.

In this book we've often recommended "body-awareness" techniques to help you monitor muscle activity. Now try a different twist—office awareness. Being alert to sources of stress in your environment can pay off in fewer injuries and a more comfortable body at the end of the day. One ergonomic chair may be worth a cartload of relaxation exercises.

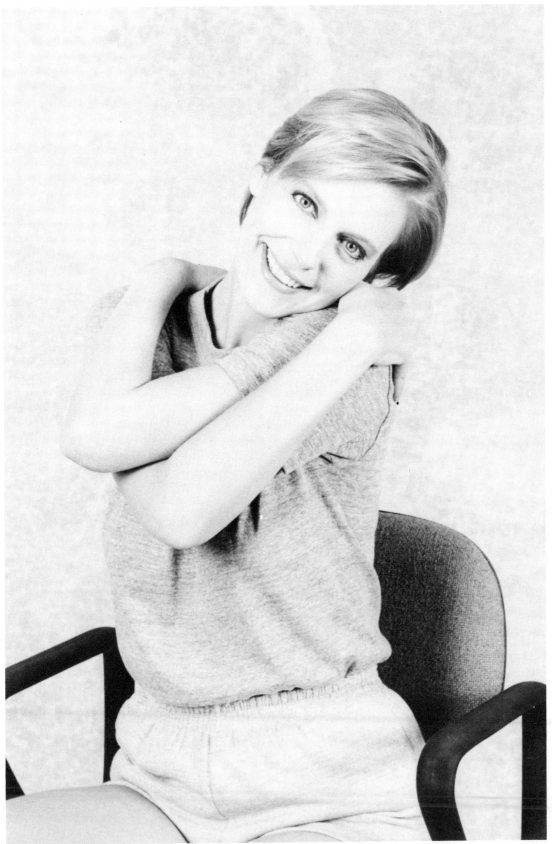

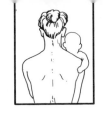

Chapter 15

A New Look at Everyday Moves

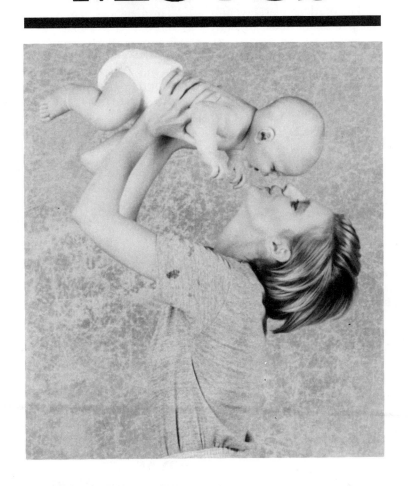

Close your eyes and visualize your body stripped down to its muscles. Now watch yourself in action: Sit, stand, climb, bend, walk—a corps of muscles endlessly contracting and flexing, synchronized in an elemental dance. Even an action as simple as standing requires the split-second tensing and relaxing of muscles that keep your bony framework erect and balanced.

But *how* you move your muscles can make the difference between feeling stiff and tense or relaxed and energetic. Most crucial to a muscle's welfare are your movement habits, those repeated patterns you rarely notice—until, finally, abused muscles sound a distress signal.

There's a great body of accumulated wisdom about how to read, diagnose, and remedy movement habits that build muscle tension. Among the leaders of that enterprise are the physicist Moshe Feldenkrais, considered a genius of body physics; Ida Rolf, who gave her name to rolfing; and F. M. Alexander, inventor of one of the first popular schools of body work.

Though these body innovators—as well as dozens of others with their own brand of body work—each developed a distinctly different therapeutic approach, they all shared a central insight: Movement habits make a subtle but critical difference in a person's efficiency, energy, and well-being.

There are now legions of muscle-and-bone workers whose craft is to remedy the fallout of poor movement habits. Though their bread and butter comes from fixing people whose movement habits have wound up in a crisis of pain, a premise of body work is that it is better to alert people to the habits that build crippling tension.

"A major problem is that we use extra muscles for activities," says body worker Gail Fries of Amherst, Massachusetts, who teaches a system of body-mind coordination. "Or we move so that the muscles that should provide primary support aren't able to, putting tremendous strain on the wrong muscles.

"It's easy to lift a five-pound weight if it's square on the palm of your hand," she adds. "But if you lift it with your fingertips, it's quite a strain. Too many movement habits create just that sort of unnecessary strain."

Movement does require that muscles tense. But the idea is to use just those muscles required for a given activity—no more. This is sometimes called "differential relaxation": You tense the appropriate muscle only to the extent the movement requires, meanwhile keeping all other muscles relaxed.

Right now, for example, as you read this, are you using muscles that waste energy and build tension? Are you fidgeting, slumped to one side, or are your head and neck projecting forward like a turkey? Are your feet tapping on the floor or your legs wrapped together in a hardworking embrace?

"The ideal way to move is to keep your body as relaxed as possible," says San Francisco body worker Roy Bonney. "For example, when sitting or standing, let your body be supported by the muscles and skeleton below, rather than by the straining of muscles from above. If your head is square atop your spine, it will be held effortlessly; if it's extended forward, your neck and shoulder muscles must contract to support it. Don't fight gravity more than you have to; it's a tremendous strain to be out of balance."

Awareness of movement habits is the first step. However, these habits are so automatic we virtually never notice them. For example, try crossing your arms. You will automatically put the arm you favor over the other. Now try it the opposite way. The first way will feel fine; the second way, strange. That's what a habit feels like—just fine.

And that's the trouble. A movement habit can feel fine and natural, and yet put unnecessary strain on your muscles. Typically, you don't notice anything until it builds a muscle knot. Even then you may not be aware of the connection.

Becoming aware of movement habits has a double advantage: It lets you change those habits that put a needless strain on your muscles; it also gives your muscles a new range of motion and more flexibility.

BODY WISDOM

One of the paradoxes of changing movement habits is that you do best if you don't try too hard—the very effort of correcting a movement can produce a counterstrain. The most effective antidote is the one that requires the least effort.

"Many people, for example, go around with their neck extended so their chin points forward, straining the neck and shoulder muscles," says·Gail Fries. "If you tell them not to do this, they'll tuck their chin down toward their neck, as though standing at stiff military attention.

"The trick is to use your awareness—rather than brute force—to correct the problem," she adds. A helpful image for correcting chin extension is the "sky hook": Think of your head as though it were hanging by a string attached at the crown of your head and extending upward to a big balloon overhead. All you need do is think of that image—without making a conscious effort to adjust your head. The image is anatomically correct. It has a life of its own that can slowly guide your head back to its best position. *You use an image, not an effort, to relax and reposition your body.*

The goal in dissolving the patterns of stress is to guide the body into movements its anatomy prefers, rather than those ordained by habit. Antidotes range from obvious changes, such as raising the height of a typewriter, to the most subtle—using a mental image as a quiet corrective.

As we go about our daily lives, the body has constant opportunity to move with ease or tension. By examining these moves, and correcting them, we can replace strain with that most salutary antidote, grace.

PATTERNS OF STRAIN

Standing

What could be simpler than standing? Yet to a body worker's trained eye, that position is fraught with subtle tension. One well-elaborated system for finding the best relationship between your upright body and gravity is the Alexander·technique. Instructors in this technique teach students to find the optimal relationship between spine, neck, and skull.

However, it's very subtle; you don't use much effort. In fact, the whole idea is to avoid effort and let your thoughts gently guide your body into a more fluid and poised way of moving. To learn more about this technique, a mainstay of many exercises in this chapter, see the Suggested Reading list on p.189. In these pages we can only give you a general idea, which goes something like this:

The mental formula to use as a suggestion to your body is: *Neck free, head up, back lengthening and widening, and shoulders spread.* You don't actually make these movements—it is just a suggestion to your body. Try this: Stand with your head lined up over your center of gravity. Think of your head floating upward a bit, pulled gently by the sky hook, and imagine your spine lengthening. At the same time, visualize having a tail growing in a downward direction. These images will help release neck and back tension, lengthen your spine, and encourage you to move with greater ease.

To help release tight muscles in the back of the pelvis, imagine you are wearing a pair of jeans with pockets at the back. See the pockets move around to the front—of your pelvis.

General Advice

The upright body is poised to move. If you must stand still for long periods, keep one foot slightly in front of the other and shift your weight from time to time. Keep your feet about six inches apart. And instead of having them parallel—a terrible position—turn your heels out a bit. Shift your foot by pivoting your heels, not your toes. This will bring your whole leg into a better position. And don't lock your knees; it will keep your legs in a more dynamic position and take the tension out of lengthy standing.

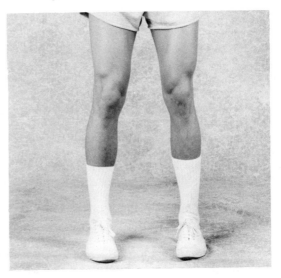

Carrying

Heavy Load

If you're carrying something fairly heavy and compact, squat and put it on one shoulder. Then stand up—keeping your back straight—and walk with it on your shoulder.

Pelvic Thrust

When you carry a heavy load in front of you—say, hugging a heavy shopping bag—your body is likely to compensate by slinging your pelvis forward, swaying your lower back. You'll be better off if you can bear the weight with your arms and abdominal muscles, keeping your spine straighter. In fact, if you can't do that, you probably shouldn't be carrying that much in the first place.

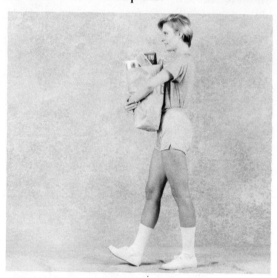

Heavy Shoulder Bag

Luggage makers did us no favor by putting shoulder straps on luggage. When carrying a heavy bag on your shoulder, you tend to tighten that shoulder in an effort to hold it up. Since we are "sided," just as we are "handed," we tend to bear loads on the favored side. If you regularly tote one-sided loads, your favored shoulder will tend to creep toward your neck. Don't be surprised if those neck, shoulder, and back muscles hurt. Switching sides is one remedy, as is supporting the strap with your hand at the shoulder. Carrying the bag in your hand, by the handle, is still better. Best bet: a backpack—but don't sling the bag over a single shoulder, or you'll run into the same problem.

Carrying a Baby

A new baby brings joy, laughter—and, too often, "mother's back." Lifting a squirmy bundle of baby from all sorts of awkward places—cribs, bathtubs, shopping carts, floor—can be a challenge. And you do it hundreds and hundreds of times.

When you lift a baby or toddler, remember to lower yourself to the child first by bending your knees. Hug the child close to you as you straighten up. And keep that back straight. No matter what the situation, before you lift a youngster, pause a moment to find the trajectory that will strain your back the least.

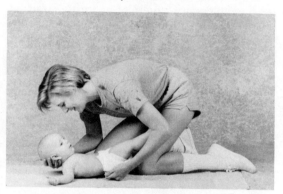

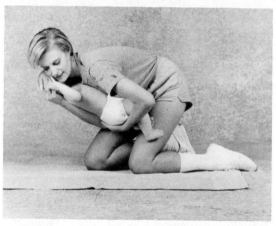

And then there's just carting the tot around the house. For young babies especially, mothers generally do well carrying the infant on one hip. But if you use the hip carry, keep your hips level, letting your arm support the baby, instead of jutting your hip out to the side. And change sides from time to time. Fathers, who have narrower hips but broader shoulders, do better with a shoulder carry. For real excursions, try a baby tote. Either method honors the basic principle: Bring baby's weight as close to your body as possible.

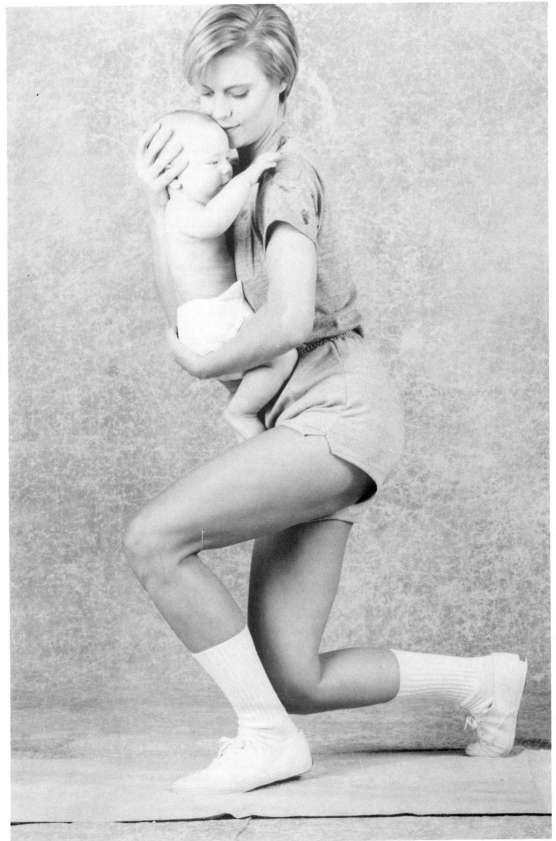

Sitting

That old saying "Sit up straight" is, of course, all wrong: The spine is never straight—it has permanent curves that were never meant to straighten out. However, you don't want to exaggerate those curves. The idea is to lengthen the spine as much as possible, within its natural limits.

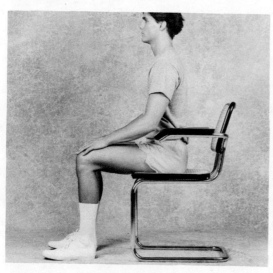

You should sit square on your "sit bones," not slumped backward on your tailbone, the bottom of the spine. The "posture of balance" is a good exercise to help you find the optimal sitting position.

Find your sit bones—the two bony protuberances in your buttocks—and balance your weight evenly on these. With your head centered along a center line of the body, imagine your head resting on an upright rod. Now imagine the sky hook—a string running from the crown of your head to a helium balloon overhead—lengthening and freeing your neck. Let your feet rest easily, flat on the floor.

That poised posture is ideal for sitting. Try to maintain it instead of slumping, scrunching, or any other favored contortion. For example, if while sitting at your desk you reach for something, try to keep your weight on your sit bones and bend from your pelvis, leading the bend with the top of your head. Bend with your whole spine, keeping your spine as long as possible during the bend. Remember: The imaginary string to the sky balloon moves in the same direction as the bend.

Walking

Of all our everyday moves perhaps none embodies our movement quirks as does walking. In this simple act we enshrine a multitude of movement patterns, including any quirks of posture.

And now again, the sky hook. That image (and the growing tail) are gentle reminders that lengthening your spine as you walk will bring your amble new grace. Think of your head leading your torso upward, your weight also ascending.

As you walk, your toes should point straight ahead. Let your shoulders hang down. Visualize your fingers brushing the ground as you walk. Let your arms swing freely.

A useful image that adds ease and balance to walking is to think of your pelvis as a level bowl full of water. Don't let it spill as you walk. This will keep your pelvis from tilting downward in front.

As you walk along, let your neck be free of tension. Don't push your head up—just think of your spine lengthening and your back widening. Let the sky hook guide you.

Lifting

As you prepare to lift something heavy, your body is likely to overprepare by bracing all its muscles. Two signs to watch for: tightening your neck and holding your breath. No matter how heavy the weight, none of this is needed.

The basics of a safe lift are determined by simple physics. Keep the object as close to your center of gravity as possible; the more you extend your back and arms from your belly and the more you bend over, the greater the load on your spine.

Get as close to the object as you can, preferably with your feet on either side of it—instead of behind it—and your knees apart. Place one foot ahead of the other, so it's already placed where you'll take your first step.

Keep your back straight through the whole lift, and use your knees to bend and straighten up. Hold the object between your legs, not out front, and use your leg muscles to lift, not your back and arms. Be sure to keep your back straight as you stand up. It may help to tighten your belly and buttock muscles as you lift.

Keep the load close to your body. If you hold the object at arm's length, it causes about ten times as much stress on your spine as when held tight against your chest or side.

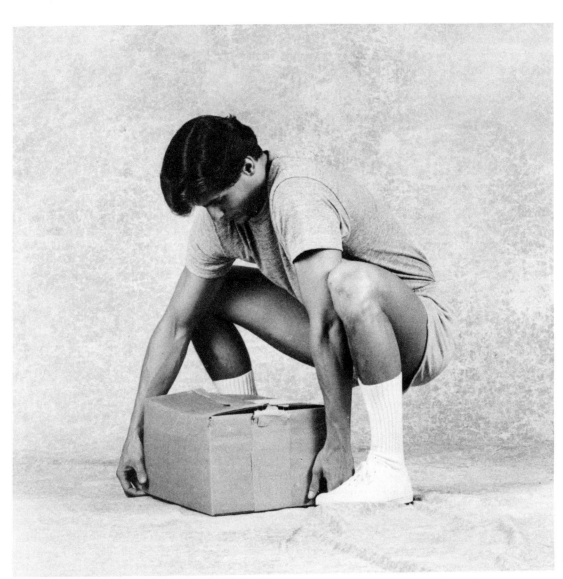

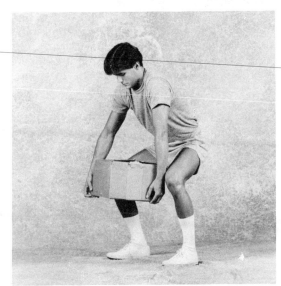

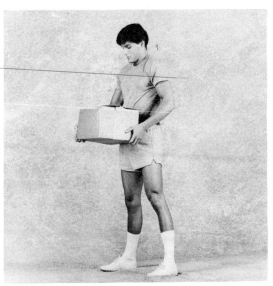

Climbing Stairs

People often trudge upstairs, using the leg that moves forward as the support leg. But it's the straight leg on the lower steps that's best for that purpose. Similarly, going downstairs, the leg that lowers to the next step bears a tremendous amount of weight. It's better to lower your body with the upper leg, rather than supporting the weight mainly with the lower leg.

A helpful image: Think of going up or down the stairs as up-and-down movement, not a forward thrust. Let your legs move you along, up and down, and let your body follow.

Driving

Driving is a special case of sitting. The trouble is that the car forces the driver to work in an odd, flexed posture, and the perils of that position are often made worse by the design of the car seat. One of the hidden costs of long drives is back pain, even for people otherwise free of back troubles.

The main deficiency in seat design is the lack of special support for the lumbar region of the lower back. The problem is worse for tall drivers in small cars; their back and knees must do a pretzel bend to fit the space.

One easy, practical fix is to place a small pillow behind the lower back. This will support the most stressed muscles.

The remedy for the overall tension of driving, though, is differential relaxation: Keep those muscles relaxed that are not involved in driving. For example, relax your shoulders and neck, two spots where driver's tension builds quickly. (See Chapter 7, "Necksavers," p.39, for some quick fixes drivers can use at stoplights. And remember to *scan*.)

If visibility is poor, as in fog, you're likely to strain forward. You'd do better to stay in your normal sitting position and move the seat forward slightly.

Working in Your Office

In the previous chapter we checked out the office furniture; here is the flip side: some tips on your personal postural habits that may get you into trouble.

Desk

For the legions whose days are spent at a desk, there are special hazards. As we have seen, a chair too low or high, or one that gives no support to the small of the back, is certain sabotage. A badly placed typewriter or computer terminal is another invitation to trouble.

In the old days clerks didn't sit at desks. They stood, or sat on a stool, at a high, inclined desk. Though it looks harsh to us today, it required a better work stance.

The modern desk is a design challenge because it looks more comfortable than it is. Points to check: Be sure your desk is at a comfortable height for you. If it's too low, you'll slump forward, a habit most of us already have, but one that should be discouraged. About elbow height is usually right for most desk work.

Desk Chair

Chairs are another major factor in your body's welfare at work. If the chair fails to give firm support to the small of your back—and most don't—get a small cushion that will. (For more on chairs, see Chapter 14, "Pain in the Office," p.159.)

Sitting up straight—that old admonition you've heard since childhood—will actually help here. But only if you do it in a relaxed way. Try it: Sit upright, with both feet on the floor in front of you. Then lower your chin slightly and lean forward, bringing both your torso and forehead gently toward the desk. Meanwhile, have the mental image of your head moving slightly upward—the sky hook—extending your spine.

Review "Sitting" in this chapter. Also, when sitting at a desk for long periods, get up and move around or do the deskercises in Chapter 14, "Pain in the Office," p.159.

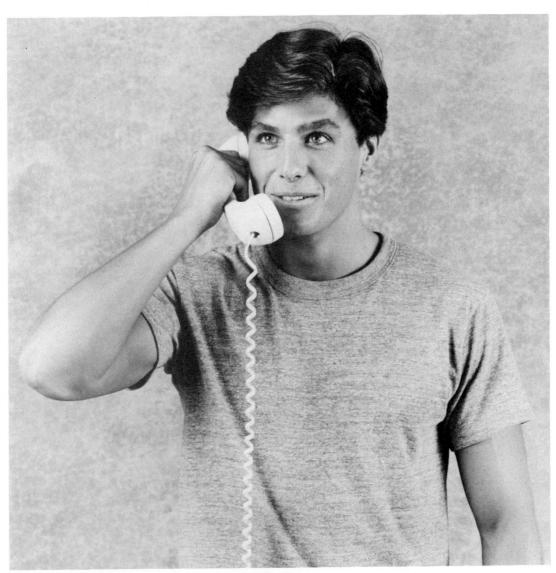

Phone

When talking on the phone, remember one principle: Move the phone to your body, not the other way around. This will counter the habit of leaning your head and neck downward to the phone and will head off the strain that habit causes.

Above all, don't hold the phone scrunched between your shoulder and ear. If your hands must be free, use a shoulder support for the phone.

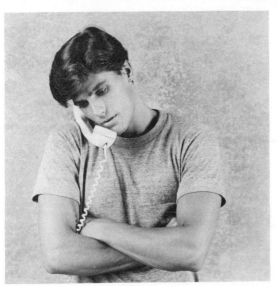

Typing

Working at a typewriter, especially for long periods, strains the neck, shoulders, and upper body, largely because your arms are extended and unsupported. Neck, shoulder, and upper-back muscles bear the weight and are subject to more tension than the mere work of typing requires.

Sitting as near as possible to the keyboard will relieve some strain. Your elbows should be even with or slightly below the keyboard—not the desk. Elbows should bend at about ninety degrees or slightly more, and the top of your thighs should clear the under side of the desk by two or three inches. To ward off tension buildup, try some necksaver quick fixes, p.66.

Reading

What's your body position as you read this? Is your spine curled forward, your head extended out toward the page? If so, you are putting a strain on the muscles that support your head and neck. If your neck and shoulders are chronic tension spots, how you hold your body while you read is almost certain to be responsible for aches.

Reposition yourself so your head doesn't hang forward and your back is upright, supported by the chair back. The main change here. is simple: Hold the reading matter up to your head; don't bring your head down to it. Try a book stand to hold the book up at a slant.

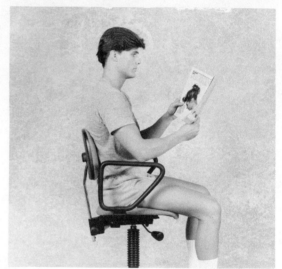

Writing

When you work at a desk, you are likely to let the desk surface define how you hold your body. That means you'll tend to bend forward over your work. Do this for a long time and you'll end up straining your neck and back.

One solution is to keep yourself upright as you write; use the sky-hook image. Your head can bend at a fifteen-degree angle without causing strain on neck and shoulder muscles. Another is to get a drawing board or architect's table that slopes up, so you don't have to bend so far to reach the paper.

For more on-the-job advice, see Chapter 14, "Pain in the Office", p.159.

Eating

Remember the phone advice? Bring the food to your mouth. The tendency to bring your mouth to the food is worst with soup. To avoid spilling, you're likely to cave in your chest, curve your neck out, and push your chin down toward the bowl. Awful!

The easiest way to eat is to lean forward slightly with your whole torso, head, and neck aligned. Your head actually seems to go up slightly as you lean. Then curl your torso a bit to bring your mouth closer when you take a bite. Let your hands and arms make the journey to your mouth. Neck and shoulders will thank you.

Gardening

Gardener's backache need not be an annual sign of spring. The amateur's enthusiasm holds a special risk because gardening often entices deskbound folks to put the body through a series of maneuvers—stooping, bending, lifting, hauling—for which it and they are ill-prepared. Some elementary cautions are in order.

First, all the standard caveats apply, especially to use your legs to bear weight when you lift or carry. But there are other tips:

■ Stooping is a big source of strain. Alternatives include getting tools with longer handles, kneeling, and sharing the muscle work by changing the hand you use.

■ Tree work, such as pruning, invites neck pain from jamming your head back while looking up, back pain from overextending your reach. Antidotes: long-handled tools, such as pruning saws; moving your ladder more often; working on a patch of the tree that's in front of you rather than just overhead.

■ Temper your ambition. Make two trips instead of one with heavy loads. The stress on your back when dumping a wheelbarrow can be immense; you may do better to empty it a bit at a time—just as you filled it. And when shoveling, don't heap the biggest load the spade will carry.

■ Digging a hole involves an especially treacherous sort of lifting, mainly because most of us do it wrong. As in all lifting, the weight should be borne by your legs, not your back. That means bending at the knees as you prepare to lift the shovel, keeping the load as close to your center of gravity as you can, and lifting by straightening your knees rather than straining with your back.

Here are some more hints:

1. Raise the load only as far as you need to.

2. Hold the shovel near the bottom of the handle, so your hand is close to the load.

3. Try to position your work so your main movement is a horizontal swing rather than a vertical lift.

4. Easy does it: small loads—and a grateful back.

Housework

The kitchen sink is potentially as dangerous as a desk. The design of sinks, particularly their height, has little to do with how the human body moves. Usually, the height is just awkward enough to encourage tension in the legs and buttocks, a hunched back and shoulders, and a shortened, tight neck straining to hold up a head leaning over to see that the dish has been scrubbed clean.

Here's a better way: Stand at the sink with your legs slightly apart, one foot slightly in front of the other. Putting one foot on top of a small stool will keep your weight from being too static. To keep your muscles from locking in tension, try moving around. Your knees should be slightly bent, your buttocks relaxed. As you lean forward, bend from your hips; don't curl your back forward.

Think of your neck and back straightening as your shoulders widen. And imagine your head moving upward in the direction your spine is pointing, while your chin brings you forward toward the sink.

Coughing

The sneeze is innocent enough; so is laughter. But if your back is prone to aches, a coughing fit can cause agony. To protect yourself from spasm:

■ When your body lunges forward, hold that position and then move back slowly. This prevents strain from yanking back quickly.

■ Tighten your belly muscles (tuck buttocks in) as you go forward, and hold them tight. You can reinforce their support by locking your fingers and holding them tight over your abdomen.

PREVENTION: STRETCHES

Use everyday situations—on the phone, waiting for a bus or on any line—to stretch your muscles, make them more flexible, and ward off knots. Hold these stretches for five to twenty seconds if possible.

Reading at Home

Lie on your back and bring the soles of your feet together, bending your knees outward and bringing your feet up toward the groin. This stretches thigh muscles.

Watching TV or Taking a Bath

Sit with your legs extended and grab your ankles—or as close to them as is comfortable.

Sitting at Your Desk

■ Reach over your head with one arm and touch the spine below your neck. Use the other hand to hold your elbow in place.

■ Reach behind your neck and clasp your hands, gently pulling upward with your arms extended.

■ Reach as high as you can with one arm, as though you were plucking oranges overhead. Then lower that arm and reach with the other. Repeat several times.

■ Put your right arm behind your back at about belly level and look over your right shoulder. Now gently twist a bit to the right. Repeat on the left side.

■ Do the clock stretches (p.68), moving your head to look at 3, 6, 9, and 12 o'clock on a huge imaginary clockface in front of you.

■ Take your shoes off and gently flex your toes; then do ankle rolls.

Sitting on the Floor

Squat instead of sitting on your bottom.

Healing Rest Position

This position requires no muscular effort and is a great relaxer. Use a firm, level surface; your bed is too soft. Lie on your back with a very small pillow under your head to maintain head-spine alignment. Bend your legs and bring your feet to rest flat on the floor, toes pointing straight ahead in line with your knees. You may wish to turn your heels out slightly so your knees rest against each other. Rest your arms across your chest horizontally with elbows on the floor. Let go and *relax*.

To get up, always roll over on your side first and use your arms to lift your body to a sitting position; then use your legs to rise to a standing position.

In leaving this chapter on prevention, try to keep the muscle ballet in mind. Movements executed with grace, economy, and a modicum of forethought leave the "performers" strong and relaxed at the end of the day. Avoid trauma in the first place and you'll have less to repair later on.

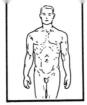

Chapter 16

The Relaxed Body

Think of your head
floating upward, pulled
gently by the sky hook.

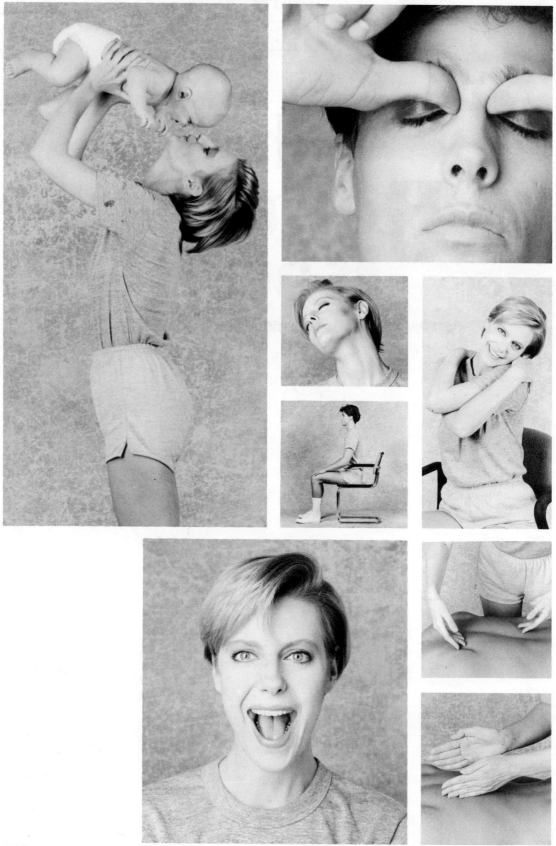

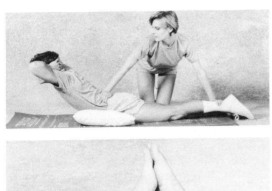

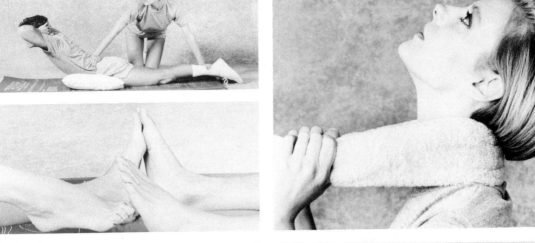

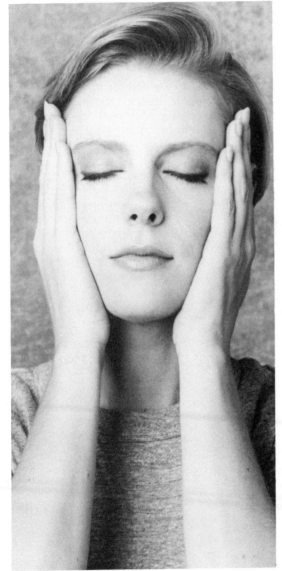

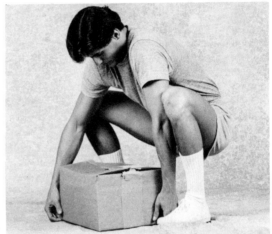

At the close of *The Relaxed Body Book*, we would like to share some afterthoughts with you on how best to put it to use. There are some basic lessons about stress to be garnered from each of the chapters, and some final principles to remember in applying the practical tips.

First, remember the mechanics of the stress spiral: Stressful moments in your day build into body tension by sneaking up on you. The trick is to use the body scan—early—to check in on your personal hot spots—the faint throb of a tension headache, muscle knots building in your neck and shoulders, early inklings of tension in your lower back, or the start of a familiar ache in your gut. Do a quick scan to tune in to those barely whispered signals, particularly on high-tension days when you're rushing around under pressure. Take a few moments to relax before misery builds.

The second point to remember is that preventing stress attacks is a daily task. Build a compatible relaxer into your schedule. The stress-style test is one way to find activities that are right for you. Whatever you choose—aerobics, meditation, muscle relaxation, or a crossword puzzle—be faithful to it. Stress prevention works best when it's part of your daily routine.

The signs of some stress problems are so subtle they can be reliably detected only by a physician. Cardiovascular disease—particularly high blood pressure—is one of these. If you recognize yourself in the description of the Type A personality, especially the quick-to-anger characteristic, you may need something more than a daily relaxer to head off heart trouble. Take seriously the advice on time management, exercise, listening to people, and cooling your temper. A lifestyle change here could save your life.

If your gut is a stress hot spot, understanding how the digestive system works offers a number of ways to prevent chronic troubles from heartburn to constipation. In general, the relaxers you choose as overall stress antidotes are also your first line of defense against gastric torment. And eating pleasantly and mindfully is an easy way to keep the digestive juices flowing happily.

When it comes to the bedroom, stress crops up in two forms: as the enemy of good sleep and the destroyer of good sex. When a stressful day ruins the mood for lovemaking, there are numerous steps you can take. One is not to worry about it too much. But if there never seems to be enough time, consider managing your schedule to make a priority of being together in a relaxed way. And once you do, sensate focus is a powerful way to attune the body to its sensuality. Then step back and let nature take its course.

As for those sleepless nights, there's a mini-catalog of do-it-yourself sleep inducers. Among them are maintaining a regular sleep schedule, avoiding alcohol, using mind-focusing methods, and even *not* staying in bed if sleep eludes you. In addition, you can choose from a range of relaxation techniques, such as autogenic suggestion, that work as overall stress inoculators but can also lull you to sleep. Good sleep and a relaxed body are soul mates. What you do for one will help the other.

In dealing with head-to-toe muscle tension, the problem and solution are the same no matter where the knot appears. When the stress spiral ends in a tense muscle, the quick fix is to restore blood flow: Apply heat and use gentle stretches and massage. If certain muscles continually go into spasm, movement and stretches are the best preventive. And give yourself a break. Take a close look at your office—or your home—to see whether you can correct despotic furniture and unfriendly equipment.

Muscle knots can also originate in your movement habits. A close inspection of routine, everyday movements, from simple standing to hauling totes and tots, may help you spot ways you inadvertently tense up. Another way to head off muscle misery is to conjure up those fanciful images that coax the body to move in harmony with its anatomical design.

And so we've come to the end of the tension trail. You've soothed, moved, stretched, massaged; you've learned to eat, sleep, sit, stand, and unwind. You know where your muscles are and can interpret their messages. You may not always have a Relaxed Body, since stress is so much a part of modern life, but you have the means to manage body tension and live closer to your relaxed best.

And now from all of us, so long, goodbye—remember to scan—and may the sky hook be with you!

RESOURCES

Suggested Reading

THE ALEXANDER TECHNIQUE
Wilfred Barlow (Warner Books, 1973)
A fine book for those who want to apply F.M.
Alexander's relaxation methods, which use the
mind to bring grace and ease to body movement.

THE AMERICAN MEDICAL ASSOCIATION
GUIDE TO BETTER SLEEP
Lynne Lamberg (Random House, 1984)
An excellent review of sleep research emphasizing
simple steps you can take to improve your sleep
and waking life.

ARE YOU TENSE?
Ben E. Benjamin (Pantheon Books, 1978)
Easy-to-use self-care techniques for releasing
muscle tension through massage and other
exercises. Provides step-by-step instructions for
deep massage.

AWARENESS THROUGH MOVEMENT
Moshe Feldenkrais (Harper & Row, 1972)
Exercises that enhance awareness of your body and
improve flexibility, by the grand master of
movement awareness.

BACKACHE: STRESS AND TENSION
Hans Kraus (Pocket Books, 1965)
The manual for backache sufferers who want to
use Dr. Kraus' techniques to prevent or cure back
problems. Features his pioneering regimen for
preventing backache.

THE COMPLETE BOOK OF SHIATSU
THERAPY
Toru Namikoshi (Japan Publications, 1981)
A well-illustrated book that presents all the
fundamental techniques plus the principles of body
structure and function that underlie shiatsu
therapy.

FOOT NOTES
Michelle Arnot (Doubleday, 1980)
A practical sourcebook offering a variety of
preventive and healing techniques for optimum
foot care.

GOOD HANDS: MASSAGE TECHNIQUES FOR
TOTAL HEALTH
Robert Bahr (New American Library, 1984)
A comprehensive introduction to the art of
massage, with an eclectic approach to whole-body
relaxation.

HEADACHE: A MULTI-MODEL PROGRAM
FOR RELIEF
C. David Tollison and Joseph W. Tollison (Sterling
Publishing, 1982)
For those who suffer from chronic headache,
advice on how to prevent or ease the pain,
including massage and movement.

KILLING PAIN WITHOUT PRESCRIPTION.
Harold Gelb, D.M.D., and Paula M. Siegel (Barnes
& Noble, 1982)
Combines theory, therapy and treatment from a
number of disciplines in a sensible program for
victims of chronic pain—headache, backache,
neck and shoulder aches, and muscular aches
anywhere in the body.

THE LANGUAGE OF THE HEART: THE
BODY'S RESPONSE TO HUMAN DIALOGUE
James J. Lynch (Basic Books, 1985)
How the process of talking and listening to others
affects the body's cardiovascular system, with
important consequences for health and well-being.
Book is based on long-term studies by psychologist
Lynch and colleagues at the University of
Maryland.

LILIAS, YOGA & YOUR LIFE
Lilias Folan (Macmillan, 1981)
Exercises, postures and relaxation techniques
adapted by a master teacher for your personal
needs—backache, sports, pregnancy, older years,
and many other special situations.

MAGGIE'S BACK BOOK
Maggie Lettvin (Houghton Mifflin, 1976)
Practical advice for those prone to back troubles.
Methods range from stretches and moves to
prevent backache to massage and other techniques
used to soothe back pain when it strikes.

MASSAGEWORKS
Lawrence D. Baloti and Lewis Harrison
(Putnam Publishing, 1983)
From Swedish to Shiatsu, an encyclopedic
collection of massage techniques.

STRETCHING
Bob Anderson (Shelter Publications, 1980)
The bible on moves that keep your muscles
flexible. Shows which stretches help what muscles,
and offers routines that protect muscles from
knots.

STRESS MANAGEMENT: A COMPREHENSIVE
GUIDE TO WELLNESS
Edward A. Charlesworth, Ph.D., and Ronald G.
Nathan, Ph.D (Atheneum, 1984)
Psychological techniques for soothing stress,
ranging from deep muscle relaxation to time
management.

Audiotapes

Progressive Relaxation/Meditation: To help break the stress spiral, *Relaxed Body Book* expert Daniel Goleman, Ph.D., guides you through two basic relaxation techniques (see Chapter 2). To order: Send $9.95, plus $1.90 for handling, to Relaxation Tape, American Health, 80 Fifth Ave., New York, NY 10011. (New York residents, add sales tax.)

Body Scan/Autogenic Suggestion: To expand your repertoire of relaxation techniques (see Chapter 2), Dr. Goleman teaches you how to do two important relaxation techniques: body scanning, which helps you monitor head-to-toe tension before it gets out of hand; autogenic suggestion, which harnesses mind power to bring peace and calm to your body. To order: Send $9.95, plus $1.90 for handling, to Body Scan Tape, American Health, 80 Fifth Ave., New York, NY 10011. (New York residents, add sales tax.)

Rest, Relax and Sleep Tape With Lilias Folan: Lilias guides you through seated relaxation, breathing, sleep stretches (see Chapter 13) and long relaxation. Send $10.95, plus $1.90 for handling, to TSI-Yoga, 800 Dixie Terminal Building, Cincinnati, OH 45202.

Organizations

The American Center for the Alexander Technique
142 West End Ave.
New York, NY 10023

Feldenkrais Guild
P.O. Box 11145 Main Office
San Francisco, CA 94101

Ohashi Institute of America (Shiatsu)
52 West 55th St.
New York, NY 10019

The American Massage Therapy Association
P.O. Box 1270
Kingsport, TN 37662

Massage Guild of California
3119 Clement St.
San Francisco, CA 94121

The Rocky Mountain Healing Arts Institute
1255 Portland Place
Boulder, CO 80302

The Association of Sleep Disorders Centers
P.O. Box 2604
Del Mar, CA 92014

The National Migraine Foundation
5252 N. Western Ave.
Chicago, IL 60625

INDEX

191

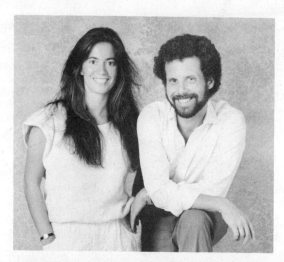

Daniel Goleman, a psychologist and a former editor of *Psychology Today*, writes regularly about behavior for *The New York Times*. While at Harvard, he did research on stress and its management and has published numerous scholarly articles on stress, meditation, and relaxation. He later spent two years in Asia studying Eastern approaches to stress management. Dr. Goleman is the editor of *The Essential Psychotherapies*, co-editor of *The Pleasures of Psychology*, and author of *Vital Lies, Simple Truths: The Psychology of Self-Deception.*

Tara Bennett-Goleman's professional background combines expertise in movement and dance, Asian awareness practices, and psychotherapy. She has led many stress-management workshops and written extensively on the subject. She is director of Creative Aging Services, a wellness program for the elderly, and co-director of Stress Management Associates in Northampton, Mass.

AMERICAN HEALTH: Fitness of Body and Mind is a health and lifestyle magazine read by over 3.7 million people. Its goal is to provide readers with the information needed to make the most of their physical and mental resources—and enjoy life to the fullest. For its lively and credible mixture of news and science-based features, the magazine was awarded a 1985 National Magazine Award for "General Excellence." T George Harris is editor-in-chief; Owen Lipstein, publisher.